Clinical Education
in Prelicensure Nursing Programs

Results from an NLN National Survey

2009

Pamela M. Ironside, PhD, RN, ANEF, FAAN

Angela M. McNelis, PhD, RN

National League
for **Nursing**

National League for Nursing
61 Broadway
New York, NY 10006
212-363-5555 or 800-669-1656
www.nln.org

ISBN 978-1-934758-11-3

Art Director, Mara Jerman

Printed in the United States of America

Clinical Education
in Prelicensure Nursing Programs

Results from an NLN National Survey

2009

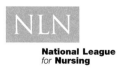

National League
for **Nursing**

Table of Contents

List of Tables vii

Foreword ix
    Theresa M. "Terry" Valiga, EdD, RN, ANEF, FAAN

Acknowledgments xi

Introduction 1

NLN Task Group on Clinical Nursing Education...2

Blue Ribbon Panel on the Future of Nursing Education Research
and Think Tank on Transforming Clinical Nursing Education 2

Background 5

Methods..6

Findings 8

    Barriers to Optimizing Students' Clinical Learning 10

    Clinical Teaching Practices 15

    Challenges to Optimizing Students' Clinical Learning.................................... 17

        Providing appropriate guidance and supervision.................................... 20

        Teaching students to "think on their feet" and
            make clinical judgments.. 26

        Providing meaningful feedback to each student 33

        Managing clinical teaching responsibilities with
            other expectations.. 37

        Supervising students' skill performance 40

Discussion 46

Limitations 54

Recommendations.. 55

References.. 57

List of Tables

Table 1 3
Members of the National League for Nursing's Blue Ribbon Panel
on the Future of Nursing Education Research

Table 2 9
Demographic Characteristics of Respondents

Table 3 11
Barriers to Optimizing Clinical Learning Experiences

Table 4 16
Most Time Consuming Instructional Activities Used in Clinical Settings

Table 5 18-19
Challenges to Teaching in Clinical Settings

Foreword

Reading the report of this national study on clinical education in prelicensure nursing programs stirred compassion for colleagues who struggle to provide clinical learning experiences for our students, helped me better understand the nature of those struggles and the near futility in managing them, and stimulated my excitement about the future we can create regarding clinical education in nursing. In this time of widespread and persistent calls for transformation and reform in all aspects of higher education, nursing seems to do everything in its power to hold on to a model of clinical education that has served us well in the past, but that may no longer be relevant, effective, or rewarding for anyone involved.

The study reported here by Ironside and McNelis tells a sobering story of the frustrations faced by our clinical faculty. It documents how exhausting such teaching is, how disappointed teachers are when they cannot give adequate attention to all students, and how time-consuming it is to help students learn how to think and to perform skills safely, as well as to give valuable feedback. Clinical educators express an inability to "do it all" and feelings of inadequacy about not being able to give their best to students. Several note how they have "learned to settle for good enough" and decided to leave their teaching positions.

Despite being quite creative in how they try to manage the many barriers and challenges they face as clinical teachers, respondents overwhelmingly reported that these strategies are only minimally or somewhat effective. In fact, only one strategy — employing graduate students as teaching assistants in the clinical setting — was reported to be effective; sadly, it was used by less than 2% of the more than 2,000 individuals who responded to this study.

These findings document what many in nursing already know — that our predominant model of clinical education "perpetuates a technical conceptualization of students' clinical experiences, which is apparent in the organization of clinical experiences in terms of required hours, checklists of the required skills to be learned and demonstrated, and the ubiquitous focus on total patient care during every clinical experience," as the authors note. It is a model that is obsolete and ineffective, and perhaps even counterproductive in the context of our current health care system.

In the midst of this reckoning, however, Ironside and McNelis offer hope and remind us of the opportunity we now have to create new models that will better serve patients, students, staff nurses, and clinical teachers. They challenge us to question — seriously and in scholarly ways — many of our current practices, such as the following:

- How do we conceptualize clinical thinking, and what do we expect of students?
- Are our questioning practices truly fostering thinking, or do they merely evaluate what students have memorized?
- Must students perform all the skills we currently expect of them in the clinical setting?
- Are some things learned better outside the clinical setting?
- To what extent do observational experiences truly contribute to student learning?
- Do our current clinical education practices truly help students become ready to transition to a practice role, and do they provide an adequate foundation for a lifetime of continued learning as a nurse?
- How can we maximize the talent and expertise of staff nurses in the clinical education process without overburdening these colleagues?

It is critical that nursing education scholars conduct rigorous research into new clinical education models, that individuals are prepared to assume roles as nursing education scholars, and that funding be made available to support such research efforts. We can no longer rely on tradition and past practice as the model for clinical education, and the data provided in this study support that assertion. The current model continues only because dedicated teachers, students, and clinical staff are willing to put on many "Band-Aids" and give enormously of themselves, but these efforts cannot be sustained. Instead, we need innovation, experimentation, and transformation; and these authors help point the way toward achieving those goals. I encourage every clinical educator and dean/director to read the report of this national survey and seriously contemplate the implications of its findings for the future of our profession.

Theresa M. "Terry" Valiga, EdD, RN, ANEF, FAAN
Director, Institute for Educational Excellence
Duke University School of Nursing

Acknowledgments

We want to acknowledge the National League for Nursing for funding this study and for their continued support of research in nursing education. We thank the 2,386 clinical faculty who found time in their hectic schedules to complete this survey. We also want to thank Sarah Zvonar for her assistance with data analyses and the preparation of this manuscript, and our many colleagues who graciously examined the survey for content and clarity.

Pamela M. Ironside is Associate Professor and Director of the Center for Research in Nursing Education at Indiana University.

Angela M. McNelis is Associate Professor and Director of Undergraduate Special Programs at Indiana University.

Clinical Education
In Prelicensure Nursing Programs[1]

Introduction

Clinical experiences are a critical part of prelicensure nursing education and are widely considered vital to the preparation of a competent nursing workforce ready and able to provide safe, quality care. Schools of nursing face persistent pressures to prepare increasing numbers of new nurses for a rapidly evolving health care system, and to do so quickly. Widespread concerns about patient safety have prompted scrutiny of prelicensure education in nursing and proposed alternatives to traditional clinical experiences. In an effort to guide the evaluation of students' clinical experiences, the National Council of State Boards of Nursing (NCSBN) reinforced the need for all prelicensure students to have "planned, structured, supervised clinical instruction across the lifespan" (NCSBN, 2005, p. 3). The American Organization of Nurse Executives (AONE) also recognized the need for structured, supervised clinical experiences and added that such experiences should be conducted by "appropriately prepared registered nurses" (AONE, 2004).

In general, it is difficult to argue that such positions are incorrect. Indeed, the discipline of nursing has long retained a commitment to providing students with clinical experience in which to learn the practice of nursing. What constitutes clinical experience, as well as the relationship between the instructional approach used and students' abilities to practice, has not been definitively documented. The lack of evidence to support pedagogical decisions about clinical education and the necessity of ensuring excellence in this critical aspect of preparation for practice prompted the National League for Nursing (NLN) to sponsor a series of initiatives to articulate current practice, propose alternatives, and study the impact of differing approaches.

---

[1] Preliminary findings from the National Survey on Clinical Education in Prelicensure Nursing Education Programs were published by McNelis, A. M., & Ironside, P. M. (2009) in N. Ard & T. M. Valiga (Eds.), *Clinical Nursing Education: Current Reflections* (pp. 25-38). New York: National League for Nursing.

NLN Task Group on Clinical Nursing Education

To articulate the who, what, where, and when of clinical instruction, the NLN Task Group on Clinical Nursing Education conducted a survey of 2,218 faculty and 28 representatives of state boards of nursing. Findings show general agreement among respondents on the "what" of clinical education — clinical education is the application of theoretical content to patient care through collaboration among faculty, students, staff, and clients (Ard, Rogers, & Vinten, 2008). Findings show a high level of agreement among respondents that students should be fully engaged in the clinical experience (99 percent) and should collaborate with faculty to identify learning outcomes and opportunities for learning (95 percent and 91 percent, respectively) (Ard et al., 2008, p. 243). Respondents also indicated that where clinical experiences occur is dependent on the goals of the course, and noted that clinical experiences should span the nursing program.

Despite widespread agreement in the discipline on the importance of clinical experiences to the preparation of new nurses for practice, very little research has been conducted to guide the design and implementation of these experiences, and little is known about the strategies that foster desired student outcomes. Ard and colleagues (2008) note that, although changes have indeed taken place in clinical education in nursing over time, these changes have not occurred as an outcome of strategic planning or rigorous study.

Blue Ribbon Panel on the Future of Nursing Education Research and Think Tank on Transforming Clinical Nursing Education

In 2006, the NLN convened a Blue Ribbon Panel of leaders in nursing education (see Table 1) to identify and articulate the priorities for future nursing education research. Among these leaders, there was strong agreement that developing and testing new models for clinical education was critically important to ensuring that new nurses are prepared for practice in contemporary health care systems. There was also recognition that new models of clinical education would require transformation of classroom teaching and the systems that support nursing teachers and students. Thus, the panel identified three major areas of focus for future research in nursing education:

1) New models of clinical education fostering partnerships between schools and clinical agencies that align clinical learning with contemporary practice and health care needs
2) Patient-centered teaching that integrates classroom and clinical education

3) Educational system redesign that supports excellence in patient-centered, integrative teaching and ongoing innovation in nursing education

A listing of the priorities for nursing education research approved by the NLN Board of Governors in 2008 can be found at http://www.nln.org/research/priorities.htm.

Table 1
**Members of the National League for Nursing's
Blue Ribbon Panel on the Future of Nursing Education Research**

Patricia Benner, PhD, RN, FAAN University of California at San Francisco San Francisco, CA Carnegie Foundation for the Advancement of Teaching Stanford, CA
Judith Halstead, DSN, RN, ANEF Indiana University Indianapolis, IN
Pamela Ironside, PhD, RN, FAAN, ANEF Indiana University Indianapolis, IN
Marilyn Oermann, PhD, RN, FAAN, ANEF Wayne State University Detroit, MI (at the time the Blue Ribbon Panel was convened) University of North Carolina at Chapel Hill Chapel Hill, NC (current appointment)
Chris Tanner, PhD, RN, FAAN Oregon Health Sciences University Portland, OR
Theresa "Terry" Valiga, EdD, RN, FAAN National League for Nursing New York, NY (at the time the Blue Ribbon Panel was convened) Duke University Durham, NC (current appointment)
Lin Jacobson, EdD, RN, CPHQ NLN Staff Liaison

Beginning with the first focal area, the NLN held an invitational think tank on transforming clinical nursing education in 2008. The purpose of the think tank was to gather nursing leaders from education, practice, and regulation, as well as interdisciplinary scholars, to explore current and emerging approaches to clinical education and the assessment of clinical performance. There was consensus among think tank members on the need to transform clinical nursing education, particularly in prelicensure programs. Members recognized that many innovative approaches and practices in clinical education were occurring at a local level, but that those innovations were not widely disseminated and their effectiveness was unknown. In addition, the factors that presented impediments to optimizing clinical learning experiences, as perceived by faculty involved in and responsible for prelicensure clinical education, had not been identified. A report detailing the work and membership of the 2008 NLN Think Tank on Transforming Clinical Nursing Education can be found at http://www.nln.org/facultydevelopment/pdf/think_tank.pdf. In response to the recommendations of the Blue Ribbon Panel and the Think Tank on Transforming Clinical Nursing Education, the NLN commissioned this national survey to examine the barriers and challenges that faculty face in optimizing students' clinical learning, the strategies they use to address these barriers and challenges, the effectiveness of these strategies, and the teaching practices faculty employ in clinical settings.

Specific survey objectives were to:
- describe faculty members' perceived barriers to optimizing clinical learning experiences for students enrolled in prelicensure nursing programs;

- identify strategies that faculty members commonly employ to address these barriers;

- document the perceived effectiveness of strategies employed to address the barriers;

- describe faculty members' perceived challenges in optimizing clinical learning experiences for students enrolled in prelicensure nursing programs;

- identify strategies that faculty members commonly employ to address these challenges;

  and

- document the perceived effectiveness of the strategies employed by faculty.

Background

Although nursing educators devote a great deal of time and energy to optimizing students' learning in clinical settings, rarely are the effects of these efforts documented via systematic evaluation or research. Indeed, in 2005 Yonge and colleagues reviewed 1,286 published articles reporting research in nursing education and found only 39 to be studies of clinical education. Without an evidence base for clinical teaching, many faculty members continue to teach as they were taught (Ironside, 2001) even though the context in which students learn and nurses practice has changed, and continues to change, dramatically. When studies are conducted, with few exceptions they involve a single class at a single school (often a class taught by the investigator), utilize small (less than 100) sample sizes (Yonge et al., 2005), and rely on anecdotal evidence or outcomes such as satisfaction that may or may not relate to actual practice abilities. In addition, this evidence is frequently collected via self-report or questionnaire (Yonge et al., 2005) rather than from observed or demonstrated practice abilities.

The paucity of research to guide clinical teaching has led to little change in the predominant model of clinical education over time. Tanner (2006a) reports that the current clinical model (one clinical faculty member assigned to a group of 8-12 students, each of whom provides care to one or two patients during the clinical experience) can be traced to the 1930s and continues to be the predominant model today.

The ubiquitous reliance on the traditional model of education continues to create problems in preparing the future workforce. For instance, this model is not easily amenable to increasing student numbers (Tobar, Wall, Parsh, & Sampson, 2007) or to providing appropriate guidance and supervision to students (McNelis & Ironside, 2009). Until recently, alternatives were often directed at changing the site of the clinical experience (e.g., service learning) or the mechanism of providing such experiences (e.g., simulation or virtual experiences) as an adjunct to the current model, rather than toward changing the overall model of clinical education itself. An unintended outcome of this failure to develop and test new models of clinical education is the continued regulation of numbers of clinical hours and faculty-to-student ratios required by specific state boards of nursing that reinforce the superiority of the current model and can inhibit the creation of promising alternatives.

One notable exception is the collaboration among the Oregon State Board of Nursing, the Oregon Consortium for Nursing Education (OCNE) (Gubrud-Howe et al., 2003; Gubrud & Schoessler, 2009), and the Dedicated Education Unit (DEU) project at the University of Portland (Moscato, Miller, Logsdon, Weinberg, &

Chorpenning, 2007; Warner & Moscato, 2009). In both of these initiatives, faculty from participating schools worked with the State Board of Nursing to substantively change the model of clinical education, prepare more students without major increases in numbers of faculty and without jeopardizing quality.

Methods

Instrument

The survey instrument was developed by the investigators. Survey items reflected insights obtained from the work of the NLN Task Group on Clinical Nursing Education, a review of the literature on clinical education in nursing, documents generated during the Blue Ribbon Panel and Think Tank on Transforming Clinical Nursing Education meetings, conversations with faculty currently engaged in clinical teaching, and the investigators' personal experience.

Survey items were organized into four sections, including both multiple choice and open-ended items. In section 1, respondents provided demographic information about their school, their role, and their experience in providing clinical education. In section 2, respondents were provided with a list of 17 barriers and asked to select and rank order the five most important barriers they faced that had hindered their efforts to optimize students' clinical learning experiences during the previous two years. For each barrier selected, respondents were asked to identify the top three strategies they had used or were presently using to address them and to rate their perception of the effectiveness of each strategy. For this survey, *barriers* were defined as "those institutional, state, or federal guidelines/policies, as well as structural, programmatic, administrative, or procedural aspects of your program/school that influence students' clinical learning and over which you personally may have little or no control."

Section 3 focused on respondents' teaching practices in clinical settings. Respondents were given a list of 13 common clinical teaching activities and asked to identify the three activities that typically took up most of their time during a clinical day, as well as to estimate the percent of each clinical day they engaged in each of the identified activities. In this section, respondents also described their use of pre- and postclinical meeting time with students, noting how these meetings occurred (with individuals or with groups), and identifying the activities that commonly took place during this time.

The fourth section focused specifically on the challenges respondents faced when teaching in clinical settings. Respondents, provided with a list of 29 common challenges, were asked to select the five most significant challenges they had faced during the previous two years and to rank order them from the most to the least challenging. Respondents were then asked to select one of their ranked challenges, identify the one most important strategy they used to address it, and rate how effective they perceived this strategy was in addressing the challenge. For this study, *challenges* were defined as "those course, context, professional, or personal aspects over which you, as a faculty member, exert some degree of control or influence or those aspects of your teaching practice that are influenced by the particular course, context or setting in which you teach and over which you, as a faculty member exert some degree of control or influence."

The survey concluded with an opportunity for respondents to add any comments about clinical teaching or evaluation that would help other nurse educators better understand the barriers and challenges to optimizing clinical learning experiences for students enrolled in prelicensure nursing programs, strategies faculty members commonly employ to address those barriers, and the effectiveness of those strategies.

Prior to release, the survey underwent rigorous pilot testing. First, members of the NLN Blue Ribbon Panel and faculty known to the investigators who had clinical teaching responsibilities across various types of programs and specialty courses reviewed an electronic copy of the survey for content, clarity, and comprehensiveness. The investigators used this feedback to refine the survey, which was then loaded onto the NLN website but not released to the public. Members of the NLN Task Group on Clinical Nursing Education participated in a second pilot testing by completing the web-based version of the survey; providing feedback on its content, format, clarity, and comprehensiveness; and reporting completion time for the survey in this format. The second testing also allowed investigators to test the ease of use and skip patterns, as well as to identify technical problems.

Procedures

Because the population of clinical nursing faculty is unknown, a convenience sample was used for this survey. Prior to launch, the membership of NLN was alerted to the upcoming survey via an announcement at the 2008 NLN Education Summit, in the October NLN Member Update, and in Fall 2008 NLN Faculty Development Bulletins. These announcements described the purpose of the study and the date the survey would be available for online completion. An email blast to all NLN members accompanied the launch of the survey and provided the URL to access the survey. This message was also posted on three listservs related to nursing education. In each message, respondents were asked to circulate the survey URL to other faculty they knew to be teaching in clinical settings, whether or not these persons belonged to the NLN. The NLN sent three reminder emails — two weeks after launch, one month after launch, and several days before closure of the survey. The URL for the survey remained open for a total of nine weeks. Response to the survey served as consent.

Sample

A total of 2,386 individuals participated in this study. Respondents did not have to be members of the NLN or teaching in a National League for Nursing Accrediting Commission (NLNAC) accredited program to participate in the study.

Findings

After approval was received from the Institutional Review Board at Indiana University, survey data were compiled by the NLN and converted into SPSS data files for transfer to Indiana University School of Nursing for analysis. Numerical data were analyzed using descriptive statistics, and qualitative data were analyzed for thematic content.

Demographics

Respondents were 2,386 faculty members, representing all 50 states. The states with the highest faculty response rates were Pennsylvania $(n = 172)$, New York $(n = 155)$, Ohio $(n = 148)$, Texas $(n = 145)$, and Indiana $(n = 89)$. In all states, faculty came from various types of institutions, with the majority teaching at a community college (35.3 percent) or a public college or university (23.5 percent) (Table 2).

Table 2
Demographic Characteristics of Respondents

Variable	N (%)
Type of institution	
• Vocational/technical	112 (4.7)
• Community college	839 (35.2)
• Hospital or medical center-based college or university	332 (13.9)
• Liberal arts college or university	138 (5.8)
• Private not-for-profit college or university	232 (9.7)
• Private for-profit college or university	118 (4.9)
• Public college or university	558 (23.4)
• Other	50 (2.1)
Type of prelicensure program offered	
• Associate	1360
• Diploma	240
• Baccalaureate	1016
Role in the school of nursing	
• Director/Dean	180 (7.5)
• Department Chair	110 (4.6)
• Program Director	102 (4.3)
• Curriculum Director	29 (1.2)
• Level Coordinator	67 (2.8)
• Course Coordinator	232 (9.7)
• Member of Curriculum Committee	15 (.6)
• Faculty Member full time	1321 (55.4)
• Faculty Member part time, temporary or adjunct	212 (8.9)
• Other	111 (4.7)
Program of primary teaching responsibility	
• Associate	1242 (52.1)
• Diploma	190 (8.0)
• Baccalaureate	882 (37.0)
Highest degree held	
• MS in nursing	1056 (44.3)
• MS in nursing with specialization in nursing education	773 (32.4)
• MS in another field	122 (5.1)
• CNE	217 (9.1)
• PhD or other doctoral degree	503 (21.1)
• Expertise in teaching via CE	199 (8.3)

Respondents were predominantly full-time faculty members (55.4 percent) teaching both clinical and didactic courses (70.8 percent). More than 16 percent *(n* = 392) were administrators (dean/director, department chair/head of department, or program director); and 13 percent *(n* = 328) worked as course, level, or curriculum coordinators (Table 2).

Types of prelicensure programs represented were associate *(n* = 1,360), diploma *(n* = 240), and baccalaureate *(n* = 1,016) (Table 2). On average, respondents had been actively engaged in prelicensure education for 12.3 years, with a range of 1 to 45 years; and more than 50 percent had been engaged for 10 or more years. A majority of faculty held a master's degree in nursing (44.3 percent) or a master's degree in nursing with specialization in nursing education (32.4 percent), and 5.1 percent held a master's degree in another field. Nearly 17 percent held a PhD, and just over 9 percent were certified nursing educators (Table 2). Table 2 provides more detailed demographic characteristics.

Barriers to Optimizing Students' Clinical Learning

In the next section of the survey, respondents were asked about barriers faced in their efforts to optimize students' clinical learning. Thinking of the course in which they had the most extensive clinical teaching responsibilities, faculty respondents rank ordered the five most important barriers faced during the previous two years, where "1" was the most important barrier faced, "2" was the second most important barrier faced, and so on. Respondents selected from a list of 17 barriers that was provided and rank ordered those they perceived to be most important (see Table 3) Results shown are the total number of respondents who ranked the given barrier as one of their top five, and thus the total number of responses to this question (11,279) exceeds the total number of respondents (2,386).

Table 3

Barriers to Optimizing Clinical Learning Experiences

Barrier	N (%)
Lack of quality clinical sites that can accommodate the number of students in my group and/or provide experiences relative to the learning objectives of my course	1218 (51)
Lack of qualified faculty	1091 (45.7)
Size of clinical groups (ratio of faculty to students)	1061 (44.5)
Restrictions on the numbers of students or limitations to students' experiences imposed by clinical agencies	971 (40.7)
Time-consuming nature of students learning multiple clinical agency systems (e.g., documentation systems are all different, hospital policies and procedures differ)	933 (39.1)
Clinical rotations now take too much time for orientation to the technology (e.g., electronic medical records, clinical information systems)	869 (36.4)
Students' inability to chart on new systems unless they are trained and certified	720 (30.2)
Rapid turnover of patients in the clinical setting	710 (29.8)
Lack of qualified clinicians to serve as preceptors	549 (23)
Unwillingness of qualified clinicians to serve as preceptors for students	519 (21.8)
Providing students with experience caring for patients with a variety of clinical conditions	518 (21.7)
Too few clinical hours in the curriculum	466 (19.5)
Lack of opportunities for effective, positive interprofessional teamwork	464 (19.4)
Acuity of patients in the clinical setting	430 (18)
Providing students with experience with culturally diverse client populations	343 (14.4)
Increased number of PRN staff in clinical settings	277 (11.6)
HIPAA restrictions limiting students' access to patient information	140 (5.9)

Data were examined in two ways, both resulting in predominantly the same findings. First, data were analyzed to determine the frequency with which the barrier was identified by respondents as one of their top five. Second, data were analyzed to determine which barrier was ranked as number one most frequently. Equal numbers of respondents (116) identified the fifth- and sixth-ranked barriers (i.e., 5 = *time-consuming nature of students learning multiple clinical agency systems* and 6 = *clinical rotations now take too much time for orientation to the technology*) as their number one barrier, although more respondents identified the former as one of the top five (933) than the latter (869). Thus, the following were the five barriers identified by faculty respondents most frequently as their number one barrier, in descending order:

- Lack of quality clinical sites that can accommodate the number of students in my group and/or provide experiences relative to the learning objectives of my course
- Lack of qualified faculty
- Size of clinical groups (ratio of faculty to students)
- Restrictions on the numbers of students or limitations to students' experiences imposed by clinical agencies
- The time-consuming nature of students learning multiple agency systems; and clinical rotations now take too much time for orientation to the technology

For each of the barriers ranked as one of their top five, respondents were provided a list of possible strategies that could be used to address that barrier. They selected up to three strategies that they used most often to address each of their top barriers and rated the effectiveness of each strategy on a 4-point scale from 1 (*not at all effective*) to 4 (*very effective*).

Lack of quality clinical sites that can accommodate the number of students in my group and/or provide experiences relative to the learning objectives of my course was identified most frequently as the number one barrier, by 544 faculty respondents, and in the top five by 1,218 respondents. The strategies most frequently used by faculty respondents to address this barrier were (1) providing clinical rotations on evenings, nights, weekends, and/or holidays; (2) substituting simulation activities for clinical hours (high-fidelity simulators, manikins, role play, videos, case studies to assist students to learn and apply clinical concepts in the context of simulated clinical scenarios); and (3) providing more observational experiences for students during clinical time. Faculty perceived these strategies to be only somewhat effective in addressing the barrier (means ranged from 2.8 to 3.2). None of the strategies used by faculty members to address this barrier were identified by respondents as very effective.

The lack of qualified faculty was the second barrier listed in the top five most frequently by respondents, with 419 indicating that it was their top barrier and 1,091 identifying it as one of their top five barriers. To address this barrier, faculty most frequently reported (1) hiring faculty with little or no preparation in teaching, (2) hiring more part-time faculty, and (3) having faculty teach overload courses. Faculty perceived that hiring faculty with little or no preparation in teaching was only minimally effective (mean 2.2); hiring more part-time faculty and having faculty teach overload courses were perceived to be somewhat effective (means of 2.9 and 2.6, respectively). None of the strategies faculty respondents reported using to address this barrier were identified as very effective.

Size of clinical groups was the third most frequently ranked barrier, with 340 respondents indicating that it was their top barrier and 1,061 identifying it as one of their top five barriers. To address this problem, faculty respondents most often reported the strategies of (1) providing more observational experiences for students during clinical time, (2) pairing students for clinical assignments, and (3) creating other kinds of learning experiences on the clinical unit to replace total patient care. Faculty again perceived these strategies to be only somewhat effective (means ranging from 3 to 3.2). The strategy that was least often used ($n = 41$) to address this barrier, but that was seen as most effective (mean of 3.5), was employing graduate students as teaching assistants in the clinical setting.

Faculty respondents ($n = 156$) identified **restrictions on the numbers of students or limitations to students' experiences imposed by clinical agencies** fourth most frequently as a barrier to optimizing students' clinical learning, with 971 faculty listing it among their top five. To address this barrier, the most frequent strategies used were (1) substituting simulation activities for clinical hours (high-fidelity simulators, manikins, role play, videos, case studies to assist students to learn and apply clinical concepts in the context of simulated clinical scenarios), (2) creating other kinds of learning experiences on the clinical unit to replace total patient care, and (3) partnering with clinical agencies (hospital's own staff helping with clinical rotations to allow experiences for students). Again, respondents reported that these strategies were only somewhat effective in addressing the barrier (means ranged from 3.1 to 3.3). None of the strategies that faculty respondents reported using to address this barrier were identified as very effective.

Simulation.

Faculty respondents who selected the strategy *substituted simulation activities for clinical hours (high-fidelity simulators, manikins, role play, videos, case students to assist students to learn and apply clinical concepts in the context of simulated clinical scenarios)* as a strategy to address a particular barrier were further prompted to estimate the percentage of clinical activities in the course provided that use simulation. Only 100 faculty responded to this question, and they indicated a range of percent usage in their clinical course. The majority (n= 56) substituted simulation activities for only 0 percent to 10 percent of the course; 35 substituted 11 percent to 25 percent of course activities with simulation, 7 substituted 26 percent to 40 percent, and only 2 substituted 41 percent to 50 percent of course activities with simulation.

Because simulation refers to such a broad array of activities, respondents were asked to specify the kinds of simulation activities they used as a substitute for clinical hours. Although only 100 respondents answered the previous question on simulation, many responded to this question on substitution. High-fidelity manikins were used by 104 respondents, medium-fidelity manikins by 78, low-fidelity manikins by 45, task trainers by 20, role playing by 95, video simulation/case study by 77, written case study by 93, and virtual or computer-based programs by 76 respondents.

The fifth most highly ranked barrier overall was the *time-consuming nature of students learning multiple clinical agency systems*, with 116 faculty identifying this as their top barrier to optimizing clinical experiences and 933 ranking it among their top five. To address this barrier, respondents reported (1) mandating preclinical orientation sessions to prepare students for the different clinical information systems and other technologies, (2) not allowing students to enter electronic data during their rotation, and (3) decreasing the number of different units/settings to which students rotate to reduce the various clinical information systems and technology that students must learn. Respondents reported that mandating preclinical orientation and decreasing the number of units to which students rotate were somewhat effective. Not allowing students to enter electronic data was perceived as minimally effective. Means were 3.2, 3, and 3.3, respectively. No strategies were identified by respondents as being very effective in addressing this barrier.

Finally, as previously discussed, 116 respondents also rated *clinical rotations now take too much time for orientation to the technology (e.g., electronic medical records, clinical information systems)* as their top barrier, with 869 indicating that it was among their top five. To address this final barrier, respondents used the same strategies as they did for the fifth barrier, namely, mandating preclinical orientation, not allowing students to enter electronic data, and decreasing the number of rotations to different units/settings. Respondents reported that these strategies were minimally to only somewhat effective in addressing this barrier, with means ranging from 2.4 to 3.2.

Although not ranked in the top five overall, barriers of technology and charting, rapid turnover of patients, lack of qualified preceptors, and unwillingness of qualified clinicians to serve as preceptors were ranked by many respondents among their top five barriers to optimizing clinical learning experiences. Although identified by the fewest respondents, Health Insurance Portability and Accountability Act (HIPAA) restrictions that limit student access to patient information still constituted a barrier for 140 faculty, indicating that this is a limitation perceived as affecting clinical learning.

Examination of strategies overall shows that none appear to be very effective no matter what the barrier. Among all strategies employed by faculty for any barrier, the most effective (M = 3.6) was using pregraduation preceptorship experiences to address the barrier of *too few clinical hours*, with 56 respondents rating this as very effective, 26 rating it as somewhat effective, and only 4 classifying it as minimally effective. The second best strategy (3.5) was using summer internships for addressing the same barrier (41 respondents rated this very effective; 18 rated it somewhat effective; 6 rated it minimally effective).

Clinical Teaching Practices

Next, the investigators probed how respondents used their time during clinical nursing education. Faculty respondents were asked to select the three activities that typically took most of their time and energy during a clinical day. Findings indicate that *supervising students' skill performance* (e.g., medication administration, IV therapy, wound care) (n = 1,636, 68.6 percent), *assisting students to synthesize clinical information and assessment findings* (n = 1,164, 48.8 percent), and *questioning students to assess their grasp of their assigned patients' clinical status* (n = 874, 36.6 percent) were the three most frequently identified activities (Table 4). After they had selected the three activities that typically took most of their time and energy during a clinical day, faculty respondents were asked to estimate the percentage of time these activities took each day. For those who said supervising students' skill performance was their most time-consuming activity, 51 percent indicated that it took between 50 percent and 100 percent of their time. For those who said assisting students to synthesize clinical information and assessment findings was their most time-consuming activity, 13 percent indicated that it took between 50 percent and 100 percent of their time; and for those who selected questioning students to assess their grasp of their assigned patients' clinical status, 10 percent indicated that it took between 50 percent and 100 percent of their time.

Table 4

Most Time Consuming Instructional Activities Used in Clinical Settings

Challenge	N (%)
Instructional Activities	N (%)
Supervising students' skill performance (e.g., medication administration, IV therapy, wound care)	1636 (68.6)
Assisting students to synthesize clinical information and assessment findings	1164 (48.8)
Questioning students to assess their grasp of their assigned patients' clinical status	874 (36.6)
Providing feedback to students on clinical paperwork/reports/recording	710 (29.8)
Ensuring safety of assigned patients	449 (18.8)
Evaluating students' overall performance	387 (16.2)
Providing feedback to students on their clinical performance	348 (14.6)
Determining students' level of preparation to provide care	314 (13.2)
Rounding on patients assigned to students in clinical group	292 (12.2)
Interacting with clinical agency staff and other health professionals	218 (9.1)
Accessing the clinical information and electronic medical records for students	178 (7.5)
Intervening when conflicts or problems arise among students, staff, and other health professionals	102 (4.3)
Charting by proxy for students in electronic systems they do not have access to	93 (3.9)

In this section, respondents were also asked about pre- and postclinical time for meeting with students. Not surprisingly, 1,834 (76.9 percent) stated that they met with students as a group prior to the beginning of the clinical experience and used this time for reviewing students' organization and priorities for the experience (*n* = 1,068), determining students' level of preparation to provide care (*n* = 1,006), and reviewing the status of patients for whom students were to provide care (*n* = 983). Only 781 respondents (32.7 percent) said that they met with students individually prior to the clinical day. Time set aside at the end of the day showed a somewhat different pattern. Almost 90 percent (*n* = 2,131) of respondents said that they set aside time to meet with students as a group at the conclusion of the clinical day and they used that time to discuss the kinds of nursing practices observed, including decisions nurses made, how nurses interacted with other health care professionals, and tasks that nurses completed (*n* = 1,591). Time was also used to have students lead discussions of the patients for whom they had provided care that day (*n* = 1,535) and for reflective activities in which students considered their experience in relation to their previous experience and that of their peers (*n* = 1,514). Respondents equally did and did not set aside individual student postclinical time. When they did, they used the time to discuss the kinds of nursing practices observed, including decisions nurses made, how nurses interacted with other health care professionals, and tasks nurses completed (*n* = 982). They also used it for reflective activities in which students considered their experience in relation to their previous experience and that of their peers (*n* = 905), as well as to review the skills the students had used and procedures completed during the clinical day (*n* = 694).

Challenges to Optimizing Students' Clinical Learning

In the final section of the survey, respondents were asked to identify the challenges they had faced when teaching in clinical settings during the previous two years. Table 5 lists the 29 items from which respondents selected their five most significant challenges. Results show the total number of respondents who ranked a challenge as one of their five most significant (10,916); again, the total number of individual respondents was 2,386.

Approximately 50 percent of faculty respondents identified *providing appropriate guidance and supervision* to each student and *teaching students to "think on their feet" and make clinical judgments* as the most significant challenges they faced in their efforts to optimize students' clinical learning. Indeed, 1,173 respondents identified *providing appropriate guidance and supervision* and 1,147 respondents identified *teaching students to "think on their feet" and make clinical judgments* as the most significant challenges they face. Respondents' identification of these two challenges as significant far exceeded that for all other challenges listed, with 15 other challenges identified in the top five by fewer than 30 percent of respondents and 12 of the possible challenges identified in the top five by fewer than 10 percent of respondents. Providing meaningful feedback to each student, managing clinical teaching responsibilities along with other expectations of the faculty role, and supervising skill performance were identified as the third, fourth, and fifth greatest challenges, respectively.

Table 5

Challenges to Teaching in Clinical Settings

Challenge	N (%)
Providing appropriate guidance and supervision to each student	1173 (50.2)
Teaching students to "think on their feet" and make clinical judgments	1147 (49.1)
Providing meaningful feedback to each student	667 (28.6)
Managing clinical teaching responsibilities with other expectations of faculty role	573 (24.5)
Supervising students' skill performance	570 (24.4)
Evaluating students' clinical performance	560 (24)
Students' focus on task completion and skill demonstration	549 (23.5)
Fostering a spirit of inquiry among students while in the clinical setting	542 (23.2)
Matching clinical experiences with classroom content	541 (23.2)
Pressure to have students "ready to hit the ground running"	492 (21.1)
Integrating learning across classroom, clinical, and lab settings	469 (20.1)
Finding ways to avoid too much student "down time"	428 (18.3)
Documenting students' learning via meaningful paperwork or assignments	400 (17.1)
Integrating new technology, such as clinical information systems and electronic health records, into the clinical experience when the school's resource centers do not have this type of system	347 (14.9)
Staying current clinically/Maintaining clinical competence and skills	304 (13)
Monitoring students in multiple agencies or on multiple units at the same time	273 (11.7)

Table 5 *(continued)*
Challenges to Teaching in Clinical Settings

Challenge	N (%)
Attending to students' attitudes toward the clinical experience	239 (10.2)
Finding ways to support overburdened staff in the clinical setting	207 (8.9)
Resistance to changing the way clinical experiences are structured	191 (8.2)
Helping students learn strategies for using resources during clinical	189 (8.1)
Fostering integrity in practice	172 (7.4)
Developing and using new models for clinical education	170 (7.3)
Helping students appreciate/understand health care systems issues	150 (6.4)
Managing differences in learning styles between faculty and students	141 (6)
Helping students understand the usefulness of their role in non-acute settings	111 (4.8)
Attending to students' attitudes toward the nursing staff	109 (4.7)
Helping students appreciate a patient's trajectory across clinical settings (e.g., acute care to home care)	94 (3.9)
Students negatively affecting the productivity of staff in the clinical agency	58 (2.5)
Attending to students' attitudes toward the clinical faculty	50 (2.1)

After identifying the five most significant challenges they faced, faculty respondents were asked to select one of the challenges in their top five and to identify the single most important strategy they had used to address it. Many respondents, however, noted how intertwined these challenges were and described a single strategy they used to address several of their identified challenges. Others enumerated specific strategies for each challenge that they identified in their top five. Not surprisingly, it was often the case that different faculty respondents described using the same strategy to address different challenges, creating a degree of redundancy among descriptions. After identifying the single most important strategy they used to address one of their top five challenges, respondents were asked to rate the effectiveness of this strategy in addressing the challenge. Overall, the strategies used by respondents were rated as only somewhat effective (mean 3.3).

The following section discusses each of the challenges that faculty respondents identified most frequently as one of the top five faced in their efforts to optimize student learning in the clinical setting, and highlights the strategies described to address it.

Providing appropriate guidance and supervision.

Many of the respondents who selected providing appropriate guidance and supervision as one of the most significant challenges they had faced in the past two years commented specifically on strategies they were using to address it. These strategies reflected three overlapping categories, those focusing on (a) the faculty member's efforts to anticipate and organize the guidance and supervision students required (e.g., "time management," "supplementing my own knowledge of the patient with information from the primary nurse," or "making a schedule" of the care activities that would require supervision), (b) the reliance on staff to provide guidance and supervision, and (c) the use of stronger and/or more experienced students to work with and supervise weaker and/or less experienced students.

Organizing the guidance and supervision students require.

Many faculty respondents commented on the importance of "being prepared" for clinical or for "prioritize[ing] instruction and skill assessment before clinical." In these cases, being prepared included anticipating students' abilities to competently care for assigned patients and devising mechanisms to provide guidance and supervision to students when this was required. As they worked through the clinical day, many faculty relied on assistive devices (e.g., checklists or schedules) or asked students to plan ahead and make "appointments" for faculty supervision when needed. Faculty respondents also relied on "investigative work" and ongoing feedback from students, staff, patients, and family members to ensure that the care being provided was timely and appropriate, as seen in this statement:

> I do a good prep on each student prior to the start of the quarter, as well as the assigned patients each week. I ask staff, the patients, and do follow-up on each student and the care provided. I ask the patient, families, [and] staff about the student's care. I get an oral report from each student with stated priorities for the care daily. I do rounds and lots of investigative work. Most of all, I get plenty of rest before clinical so I am sharp and ready to take on the challenges of 7 students in the clinical setting.

Even when they were prepared, though, the overwhelming demands of organizing the guidance and supervision that students needed were central to many respondents' comments:

> With a group of 7 or 8 students (the groups are now routinely 8), it was very difficult to pass multiple meds with each student and assess whether they were prepared to do so. I either had to find a way to do it, or not let half the group pass meds, which hindered their learning and clinical experiences — same thing with other clinical tasks such as sterile dressings, tube feedings, etc. Students want to have hands on experiences, and it does help to allow them these tasks, provided I have time to help them see the total picture and not just the task itself. However, I can only be in one place at one time, so my ability to work with the students individually was limited at times.

> I stay very busy, always accessible, stay on the unit at all times, do not take lunch break. Very organized, have lots of "check-off lists," ask students lots of questions, major multitasking.

Another respondent stressed the importance of being "incredibly organized," maintaining clear communication with students and staff, and guiding students to "pull it all together."

> It has helped to be incredibly organized with patient assignments, making it very clear with staff what students will and won't be doing for patients, so there is no room for misunderstanding about this, making rounds many times each day to check on how each student is doing and what they need help with, and pulling it all together in post-conference for shared learning. No wonder clinical teaching is so exhausting.

Many participants also noted how "exhausting" the demands of organizing the guidance and supervision needed by students were, particularly given the acuity of patients and the number of students in each clinical group. Some respondents indicated that their school was decreasing enrollment or hiring new staff or teaching assistants (graduate or baccalaureate prepared) to assist with supervision. Many more described providing "observational" experiences for students to decrease the number of students for whom guidance and supervision were required, limiting the skills students used during the clinical day (e.g., "limit[ing] medication administration and treatments to only half of the students on a clinical day"), or limiting the interactions they had with students during the clinical day (e.g., "[I] try to limit my time, giving 30 minutes to each student/day.")

Just as commonly, however, respondents expressed frustration and a sense of futility about not being able to offer the kind of guidance and supervision that they believed students needed and that they thought they should provide ("I'm still trying to figure out how to be everywhere at once"). In other words, respondents frequently commented that there was not enough time to provide guidance and supervision to students.

> Honestly, no matter what I did, I never had enough time to spend quality time with each student to facilitate the levels of integration and critical thinking that I would have liked. My biggest challenge… was a lack of time. Or, in other words, I had too many students all wanting me to come "watch" them. I could not in good conscience abandon them to skills on their own — that would be unethical and unsafe practice, nor did I feel I could abandon them to the nurses on the units — they were already too busy anyway. So, every day I run my butt off to spend as much time with as many students as I can. But it is not enough. It is not the quality I wish to provide. And so every day I go home feeling like I was not able to give my best to my students.

> I work very hard in the clinical area with little to no down time. I do what I can do and realize with 10 students on multiple units, that is the best that can be done. I have worked to change the 10 to 1 student/teacher ratio, but our state board of nursing, while acknowledging 10 to 1 is too many, [has] not been willing to change the ratio.

Few would deny that *providing appropriate guidance and supervision* is imperative for students' learning in clinical settings where the margin of error is small and the potential consequences of error are, at times, extreme. It is noteworthy that faculty respondents so frequently described their persistent attempts to provide this guidance, even in difficult or overwhelming situations, by better organizing themselves and/or the work that had to be completed. On one hand, this approach is important in that nurses commonly practice in difficult and overwhelming situations; so these efforts can be viewed as a mechanism through which faculty can role model an important skill that new nurses need in order to safely enter practice. On the other hand, the frequent reference to the exhausting nature of this work and the frustration and futility experienced by faculty may be a harbinger that, at least in many cases, the limits of personal organization have been reached and the *provision of appropriate guidance and supervision* of students in many clinical settings is in jeopardy. Nonetheless, the ethical need to keep both patients and students safe during the clinical experience pervaded respondents' practice, often leading faculty to solicit assistance from others to supervise students' practice.

Reliance on staff nurses and preceptors.

To deal with the demands of providing appropriate guidance and supervision to students during clinical experiences, many respondents cited relying on staff nurses "to be an extra set of eyes" or to be preceptors working one-on-one with students "to ensure that [each] student is monitored." Respondents frequently noted the importance of developing "good relationships" with staff nurses so that students' experiences were not compromised and staff nurses were not overburdened.

One method [to *provide appropriate guidance and supervision*] is to develop a good relationship with staff nurses so that they know what you expect of your students and they can be another set of eyes for you. Getting to know them also helps you decide which nurses you can trust for appropriate guidance.

Developing effective and trusting relationships with staff nurses on unit enables me to assign students to these trusted colleagues for guidance with my stronger students while I work with the weaker students.

I need to rely on nurses who are willing to help students when I'm with another student on one of the four units on two floors. They are great, but it does add to their workload, and I feel like the best ones may burn out! Occasionally, the students need to observe things that they could do with me present but that the RNs just don't have time to supervise if I can't get there.

Providing appropriate guidance and supervision to each student is the most significant challenge I face as a clinical instructor on a busy medical-surgical unit. The professionals I work with are the only things that make this challenge bearable. We have developed, over the years, a healthy respect for each other's burdens and when I am busy with a student the staff will take the time to supervise the absolutely essential tasks the students have to perform for the patients these professionals are caring for during the whole day.

Importantly, some participants noted the reciprocity that good relationships with staff fostered for both students and staff.

The staff [nurses] assist me with monitoring students during clinical rotations (e.g., medication administration, dressing changes), provide constructive feedback and help to seek out appropriate experiences (e.g., new procedures such as IV starts, etc.). The students also support the staff by assisting on the unit when ancillary help is not available by answering phones, taking vital signs, re-stocking equipment and linens, etc.

Although some respondents mentioned staff who were resistant to working with or even hostile to students, the majority noted how the provision of appropriate guidance and supervision to students relied on their fostering good working relationships and clear communication with staff nurses. Through these relationships, respondents were able to rely on staff nurses they "trusted" to "share the burdens" of teaching, learning, and practicing nursing in busy clinical areas.

The reliance on staff nurses to *provide appropriate guidance and supervision* to students in clinical settings is certainly nothing new. Indeed, historically, clinical education was the purview of staff, and students were expected to assist staff or independently complete the work assigned or delegated. The limitations of this apprenticeship model have been well documented, and there is widespread consensus in the discipline that the emphasis in students' clinical experiences is learning and not staffing the clinical unit.

The comments provided by respondents in this study indicate that *providing appropriate guidance and supervision* requires faculty and staff nurses to work together to keep both students and patients safe. Certainly the acuity of patients and the complexity of current health care settings make it prudent for more than one person to supervise students as they learn to provide care. This is a common practice in nursing, and nurses consistently rely on backup from their peers (and others) in the provision of care. Indeed, Luhanga, Yonge, and Myrick (2008) note the importance of staff nurses in monitoring unsafe practice during student experiences.

What is not clear, however, is if and how the guidance and supervision provided by staff nurses merely fills the gap in supervision or intentionally contributes to students' learning. In other words, does the supervision provided by staff nurses when a faculty member is not present merely serve as an opportunity for a student to complete a skill that he or she cannot do independently, or does the staff nurse foster and support a broader view of clinical learning by helping students to notice and respond to patients' concerns or subtle changes in status, as well as to think critically about the care being given within the larger system of care? Does the reliance on staff nurses to *provide appropriate guidance and supervision* give students an opportunity to build effective relationships with expert nurses that enable exploration of the nuances of clinical situations and the possibilities for care that could be enacted in any given situation? The sheer frequency of the practice of relying on staff nurses to guide and supervise students makes this an important area for future investigation.

Use of students to provide guidance and supervision to other students.

In addition to devising ways to organize and prioritize their time and relying on staff nurses to *provide appropriate guidance and supervision* to students during clinical experiences, many respondents spoke of using other students in supervisory roles. In some cases, respondents shared how experienced students (often seniors in a leadership/management course) supervised students not as far along in the program, whereas others described rotating students through team leading or management types of roles in which one student provided supervision to other students in the clinical group. Respondents deemed such experiences beneficial both to the students supervising and to the students being supervised in that they helped students to appreciate broader, systems issues influencing care, including skills such as delegation and communication, as well as enhancing their ability to provide appropriate guidance and supervision to all students.

Equally common were respondents' accounts of pairing students to provide care to assigned patients. In some cases, this strategy was employed to limit the number of patients for whom the faculty member was responsible (e.g., "early on I pair students to reduce the number of clinical situations we are involved in so that I can focus better on the situations I am working in") and, because students were working in dyads, the number of students that faculty needed to guide and supervise (e.g., "I buddy up the students so 2 students are assigned to 1 client [so] I can supervise two students at the same time allowing me to provide more guidance"). Many respondents, however, also related how pairing presented opportunities for students to guide and supervise each other.

> I have been pairing students up, or allowing another student to watch a classmate perform a skill, and then allow the student watching to critique the skill and ask if that person would have done anything differently. I think that helps them see different viewpoints or other ways of doing things.

In addressing the challenge of *providing appropriate guidance and supervision* to students, a number of respondents shared that this challenge required a variety of strategies, and their descriptions frequently included several strategies that had been implemented simultaneously to address it. Other respondents described strategies that they had tried unsuccessfully (e.g., "I have tried several solutions but none permanent or lasting") or shared that they had "not really found a way to address this [challenge]."

Clearly, many of the strategies that faculty respondents reported using to address the challenge of *providing appropriate guidance and supervision* to students hold promise for optimizing students' clinical learning experiences. For instance, pairing students may indeed promote safety competencies such as teamwork and collaboration and reducing reliance on memory (by enabling students to consult with a peer or to discuss alternative approaches to a given situation) (Cronenwett et al., 2007). It may also provide students with opportunities to engage in and become more skilled at peer teaching (Aston & Molassiotis, 2003; Daley, Menke, Kirkpatrick, & Sheets, 2008; Secomb, 2007). Certainly, pairing students does decrease the sheer number of patients for whom a faculty member is responsible and thus the number of skills, procedures, or interventions to be supervised, allowing faculty members to provide more guidance and supervision before, during, and after care delivery. Neither the impact of these strategies on the quality of care provided on a unit nor the effectiveness of these strategies in promoting students' learning and readiness for practice has been demonstrated; and these issues remain priorities for research. In addition, patient perceptions of receiving care from pairs or groups of students warrant further investigation.

Teaching students to "think on their feet" and make clinical judgments.

In addition to *providing appropriate guidance and supervision* to each student, an overwhelming number of respondents identified teaching students to *"think on their feet" and make clinical judgments* as one of the most significant challenges faced, and many commented on the strategies they used to address it. These strategies most commonly included the use of various ways of questioning students, providing simulated experiences or case studies that mimic complex clinical situations, and engaging students in learning activities outside clinical that required them to reflect on their practice experiences (often during postclinical conferences) or to represent their practice knowledge conceptually.

Questioning.

By far the most common strategy that faculty respondents reported using to *teach students to "think on their feet" and make clinical judgments* was questioning (recall that in the previous section that only 10 percent of faculty respondents who identified this as the most time-consuming strategy indicated that it accounted for more than 50 percent of their time in clinical settings). Some respondents identified the use of particular questioning strategies, such as "a Socratic approach" or the "5 why method," whereas others reported asking more general "what if" and "what next" questions. Some respondents characterized questioning as a means to *evaluate* students' thinking and judgment (e.g., "I use a lot of questioning during preconference in determining students' knowledge of their plan of care for the day") rather than as a means to *teach* thinking and judgment.

It was noteworthy how often respondents stated that they used questioning "constantly" or "continually" or referred to "quizzing" students, "always responding to a student's question with a question," and "not giving [students] answers." This type of questioning could happen "anytime and anywhere in [the] clinical setting" and could continue "until there are no questions left unanswered."

In contrast, other respondents more clearly emphasized their efforts to use questioning as a way to help students "connect the dots," "see the big picture," or explore possibilities for care ("so what are you thinking about this?"), as well as to help them see what was (and was not) working in the current approach to providing care.

I use statements starting with "I wonder . . . if we did XYZ what would that look like?" [I have] students "imagine" along [which] helps them learn to think. Some students need more coaching than others, but they all get the hang of it eventually!

[I] give [students] "what ifs" and work through the options that are available, what they would choose and why. [I] discuss the ramifications of the decision they made and discuss what might have happened if they had chosen a different option.

I spend a lot of time asking questions. Why this? Why not this? And helping them to make connections… what do you think about this and this? How does this fit with X?

Making rounds was another strategy respondents commonly identified that helped them "focus on critical thinking skills and judgment" and "hear [students'] thinking" during a clinical experience. Others focused on "thinking out loud" activities during pre- and postclinical conferences or during conferences planned midway through the clinical experience when students were away from the clinical unit and able to focus more on "thinking together" and "seeing the whole picture."

Importantly, some respondents specifically pointed to the importance of creating a safe environment for questioning as a way of fostering students' abilities to *"think on their feet"* and make clinical judgments.

I have addressed [the challenges of *teaching students to think on their feet and make clinical judgments*] using a prompting questioning style — asking them to think and providing them a safe environment to be wrong.

My students know that they must be able to answer "why" to everything they do. Some are reluctant to do this at first because they fear they will be wrong. When they realize there is no penalty for thinking, they are more likely to try to figure out the response to my frequent question, "WHY?"

…I let the students know that I will be asking them to… link pathophysiology to signs and symptoms, meds, etc. I assure them that I do not yell at them, rather lead them on the path to "make the puzzle pieces fit together" or "connect the dots."

Other respondents also noted the importance of using questioning in a group setting ("[so] other students can chime in, so the student [being questioned] doesn't freeze up"). In these cases, the emphasis of the interaction between teacher and students was on questioning as a strategy for "thinking through" or "talking through" clinical experiences. Several respondents noted that teaching thinking was particularly "time-consuming," as well as being a "difficult skill to learn," one that "takes time" to develop. In most cases, more experienced faculty were resources for improving this aspect of clinical teaching. One participant noted,

I am new to this [clinical teaching] so [*teaching students to "think on their feet" and make clinical judgments*] is a challenge for me at this point. I am trying to find out what works, but right now it is trial and error. Asking other more seasoned faculty how they handle this has been my strategy in addressing this issue.

Clearly, faculty respondents recognized the importance of questioning students who are learning in clinical settings. Faculty do have an obligation to assess students' knowledge, skills, attitudes, and plan of care before students provide care to an actual patient. This is a very narrow use of this strategy, and research has documented that such questioning may not promote thinking as much as it prompts the recall and recitation of information memorized during preparation for clinical (Ironside, 2005). In fact, the effectiveness of barraging students with questions as a way to teach (or evaluate) thinking is suspect and warrants further inquiry. Due in part to the low levels of pedagogical literacy among current faculty members, the lack of preparation for teaching among current faculties (as well as staff nurses and preceptors), and new faculty members' reliance on "seasoned faculty," the overuse of this strategy to merely document or verify a student's preparation in the guise of teaching thinking persists.

New pedagogies that foster multiperspectival thinking (Ironside, 2006; Scheckel & Ironside, 2006) hold promise for extending disciplinary questioning practices. That is, new pedagogies can help students explore possibilities for listening and responding to clinical encounters (Diekelmann & Diekelmann, 2009), imagine alternatives for care, and anticipate outcomes in the specific context of practice (Benner, Sutphen, Leonard, & Day, 2009). Perhaps we don't talk enough, as teachers, about the ways in which we use questioning and the effect of our questioning practices on students' learning, thinking, and emerging practice.

Providing simulated experiences or case studies.

As with many of the other challenges faculty identified as significant, when describing strategies used to *teach students to "think on their feet" and make clinical judgments* they very commonly mentioned the use of simulated experiences or case studies that mimicked complex clinical situations. They frequently cited high-fidelity simulation scenarios as a strategy used to prepare students for clinical by providing time to practice necessary skills and decrease students' anxiety.

> [We] utilize the human patient simulator to do open lab sessions to practice the role of the nurse with changing patient scenarios. This is above and beyond the scheduled clinical time.

> Getting students to think on their feet, when they are nervous, is difficult. We run simulations before they get to the hospital, this makes them less nervous in the hospital.

At other times, faculty used simulation to help students practice thinking about the care required by complex patients. For instance, some respondents spoke of "adding high fidelity simulations which *require* clinical judgments" (emphasis added), while others made comments like "the use of simulation has helped tremendously. Using SIM man we are able to ensure that the students see complex patients in a controlled setting."

> [We have the students] practice clinical simulations (similar to ACLS/PALS) and clinical scenarios in which the student is expected to assess the client

condition and make a clinical judgment, respond appropriately, provide appropriate nursing care, delegate, etc.

It was noteworthy that only one respondent mentioned using simulation in place of actual clinical time to *teach students to "think on their feet" and make clinical judgments* even though this was the strategy that participants most frequently reported using to address the barrier of *restrictions on the numbers of students or limitations to students' experiences imposed by clinical agencies*.

We have assigned each student 33 percent of their clinical lab time in the HPS [human patient simulation] Learning Lab. We call our lab "Caring Hands Hospital" and it is treated as an actual clinical learning experience. We have faculty who now can manage the lab and know how to make it a "reality based" learning experience. We make certain the students are exposed to challenges in the HPS Lab and then allow them to learn more during the debriefing session at the end of the learning module.

Clearly, simulation is a common strategy that faculty employ to *teach students to "think on their feet" and make clinical judgments*. The literature supporting simulation to foster particular skills (e.g., clinical judgment), to provide opportunities for practice and making mistakes in a safe setting, and to allow faculty to standardize the assessment of particular knowledge or skills is growing rapidly. Simulation is unique in that it frequently removes the instructor's direct guidance at the bedside, allowing students the opportunity to make independent nursing decisions in a safe environment where cues can be provided. Although the use of high-tech manikins was frequently mentioned, faculty respondents' descriptions also pointed to low-tech strategies to mimic clinical situations for the purpose of teaching thinking. Though there is great enthusiasm for the potential of a wide variety of simulation strategies to assist students to learn the practice of nursing, the extent to which these experiences are equivalent to, better than, or worse than learning in actual clinical settings (so that clinical time can be replaced with simulation) remains to be documented. Moreover, simulation was often described in the context of practicing necessary skills and decreasing students' anxiety even though the relationship of these outcomes to teaching thinking and making clinical judgments has not been demonstrated. Research examining the relationships among these constructs in the context of nursing practice is needed.

Engaging students in learning activities outside clinical.

Interestingly, many of the strategies that faculty respondents reported using to address the challenge of *teaching students to "think on their feet" and make clinical judgments* were strategies used outside the clinical experience. Frequently these strategies were linked quite directly to clinical learning (e.g., "[I] use simulation learning, case studies, and role playing to help students think in situations and evaluat[e] the outcome of the situation"), whereas at other times the link to clinical learning was not as clear (e.g., "I have used case studies from beginning to end in the classroom and all our lectures are pre-recorded").

The strategies described to *teach students to "think on their feet" and make clinical judgments* spanned students' experience or level. At times, case studies were used as a way to help more experienced students "recap" what they had learned throughout the program or to practice management skills. Other respondents stressed the importance of postclinical conferences or "debriefing" that occurred after the simulation as helpful to less experienced students:

> I teach freshman so [*teaching students to "think on their feet" and making clinical judgments*] happens more in conference or debriefing settings where I can have them imagine other ways their day could have gone and how they would have handled things differently based on different client response. I also try to change the context of care to help them see how their nursing response would change.

Assisting students to reflect on their experiences in practice during faculty-student conferences or via journaling provided another opportunity for respondents to *teach students to "think on their feet" and make clinical judgments*. At times this reflection was highly structured (e.g., "concept cards"), at other times less so.

> [I] allow some time of thought and reflection and discussion of possibilities and what is best for that one particular patient versus another.

> I continually pull prior experiences into play, reinforce prior interventions (successes and failures), developing themes, relating personal stories and experiences.

In the context of the strategies faculty use to *teach students to "think on their feet" and make clinical judgments*, the use of some mechanism for students to document their thinking related to the care being planned or provided was evident, although again the link between documenting and teaching thinking was not clear.

> I require the students to complete concept maps to prepare for patient care.
> Then we discuss how health status, meds, and interventions are related *as time*
> *allows* during the shift [emphasis added].

> We have implemented the use of concept maps in lieu of the traditional
> 6-column form for care planning. This ability to graphically view their
> patient's condition and be able to easily modify it during the day of care has
> helped [address this challenge].

For these respondents, the depiction of various aspects of care via a concept map appeared to be the salient feature that prompted students' thinking (e.g., discussion occurred as time allowed rather than as a central feature of the strategy). Other respondents more clearly described moving away from this approach to better guide students' thinking.

> [We] eliminated most of the "care plan" component of paperwork and
> changed to focused activities for better understanding of the clinical picture
> of each patient. Looking more at what is critical to know, nice to know, or
> can be looked up in a reference and using that hierarchy to guide information
> and activities presented.

> I replaced care plans and I am now focusing on the student looking at the
> larger health care system and how the patient fits into it. For example, the
> student has to use Patient Safety Goals to assess the environment of their
> patient.

Faculty respondents described many strategies that they employ to *teach students to "think on their feet" and make clinical judgments*, and the brevity of their responses presents significant limitations to understanding the full extent of how these strategies are used. Nonetheless, somewhat troubling is the underlying tension between strategies that provide mechanisms for students to document (and faculty to evaluate) their thinking and those directed toward fostering students' abilities to "think on their feet" or "think like a nurse" (Tanner, 2006b).

In addition, the assumption that there is a clear, direct, and corresponding relationship between learning that occurs outside the clinical setting (in classroom or lab or during preparation for clinical) and the use or application of that learning in actual clinical experiences has not been well documented. It would be timely to reconsider the common conceptualization of classroom learning as "theoretical," occurring before and informing clinical (Benner et al., 2009). Research investigating the relationships between "where" students learn and "what" is learned would assist in the creation of more seamless approaches to teaching the practice of nursing. It may also be the case that the difficulty respondents had in clearly describing the strategies they used to *teach students to "think on their feet" and make clinical judgments* is related to the disparate ways of conceptualizing critical thinking in the discipline, and thus what faculty are actually trying to promote with these strategies may vary as widely as the strategies themselves.

Providing meaningful feedback to each student.

Nearly 25 percent of faculty respondents identified *providing meaningful feedback to each student* as one of the five most significant challenges, and 74 respondents identified it as the most significant challenge they faced in optimizing students' clinical learning. Though fewer faculty shared the single most important strategy they used to address this challenge than for the top two (previously described) challenges, many innovative approaches were offered.

Not surprisingly, many respondents described their efforts to meet with students individually either during ("I make it a point to talk with each student during the day about their patient") or after the clinical experience ("I also find it helpful to meet with students individually outside clinical to discuss significant issues"). At times, these one-on-one conversations involved providing feedback relative to the faculty member's evaluation of the student's performance. At other times, this feedback was directed toward the integration of classroom material and clinical experiences.

> I address [*providing meaningful feedback to each student*] by taking time one-on-one with each student, by reviewing prior paperwork, asking questions regarding patient selection for the day, and going over specifics of the chart and other clinical information with the student. Asking questions and relating to classroom content. This is very time consuming but worth it for each student's learning in my clinical groups.

Though spending one-on-one time with students was clearly a goal of most faculty respondents, many emphasized how time-consuming this was (e.g., "It commonly takes me 1.5 hours to grade each student's paperwork and 2+ to grade those students who are really struggling."). Several respondents had worked out in detail the time involved in providing meaningful feedback.

I find that I have very little one-on-one time with [students] in a setting where we can actually discuss pertinent issues. I have a 10-hour clinical day. If I subtract 1 hour for post conference and 1.5 hours for lunch, potty breaks and running from unit to unit (my students are scattered among 4 units), that leaves 7.5 hours. If I divide 7.5 by 10 that leaves a total of 45 minutes to spend with each student to meet all of their needs, including med passes and supervising other skills.

Providing meaningful feedback as a component of clinical performance evaluation requires verbal feedback in the clinical area as well as timely, written feedback following the clinical experience. At the conclusion of each clinical day I provide written feedback for each student on clinical performance and the required written work for the course. This is time intensive (i.e., 30 minutes-60 minutes per student). The students are required to read, comment, and sign each daily performance narrative. These daily narratives become part of the midterm and final evaluation clinical performance document in support of performance ratings. While time consuming, this method of documentation is helpful to support trends in excellent as well as poor performance especially if performance results in a clinical failure. Sadly compensation for clinical teaching is less than [for classroom faculty,] so while this strategy benefits student learning and performance the cost of time for faculty is not reflected in compensation nor are other expectations of the faculty role adjusted. This becomes a driving force for consideration of a return to clinical practice.

Occasionally, respondents shared school wide efforts to enhance the feedback provided to students ("keeping instructor to student ratio at 1 to 6 instead of 1 to 8 has helped with evaluating clinical performance and providing feedback," and "reducing size of clinical groups from 8-9 to 6-7"). To deal with the time-consuming nature of providing meaningful feedback, some faculty respondents wrote about setting small goals for the amount of time they would spend with each student to provide feedback (emphasis added in each instance):

[I] spend *ten minutes a day* with each student discussing their performance.

I work to meet individually with each student *at least once* during the 6-hour day.

I try to be cognizant of my lack of feedback and give feedback to *at least one student* each clinical day.

I accept that it is not possible to divide my time with the students equitably, so I attempt on my next clinical day to spend more time with students I was unable to be with on the previous clinical day.

More often, however, descriptions referred to increased use of technology (e.g., "discussion boards," "e-mail," and "computerizing our feedback form") to provide meaningful feedback at a distance.

[I] use online journaling about the clinical experience. I ask the students to do this immediately after each clinical and I try to get feedback to them before the next clinical. By writing online, they tend to expand on their experiences more and this gives me a better picture of what really went on — given the fact that I cannot be in every room with eight students. It also helps encourage reflection. I believe that a great deal of the learning comes during this reflection and I can build on the students' [comments regarding] "what I would do differently if I had the chance to rewind today."

[We] have implemented reflective clinical journaling by e-mail to provide more prompt faculty response to student clinical experiences.

We are trying to develop electronic methods as well as "standardized" statements to accommodate feedback.

We teach at a distance and most conversations happen via phone or electronically.

If I do not have time to give fact-to-face feedback, I send them an e-mail.

Many faculty shared efforts to "revise paperwork to be shorter" or to "develop meaningful rubrics" more closely linked to course objectives in order to provide meaningful feedback. As with the strategies described to address other challenges, some respondents reported cutting down on the skills they must supervise to allow more time for providing feedback.

I have tried to meet with students individually at the beginning of clinical rather than as a group to offer feedback on paperwork, prep, etc., and then I also have limited the number of students administering meds on any one day so that I can spend more time with everyone as this takes the majority of my time on the unit. I (and they) do not feel as rushed and I am able to offer more feedback during our time together rather than rushing off to yet another task, skill, [or] med administration.

Faculty respondents also described strategies they had developed to engage students more fully in the feedback process though self- or peer-evaluation.

Rather than grading the student's papers alone, I have the students review their papers with me and discuss their work. This seems to help them feel more accountable for their work, more comfortable in asking me questions or accessing resources before handing their work in, and better able to identify their own strengths and areas of potential improvement. I find it much more effective to directly ask a student to clarify their work, than to ask the same question in written form.

[I] had students grade their own paperwork using my grading guide; then [I] graded the same paperwork giving written feedback on what they missed.

[I'm] having the students set their own learning goals in addition to my expectations, and then regularly writing in their reflective journal about same. Finally, having them do a final self-evaluation, prior to our discussion.

Students submit a weekly electronic journal addressing goals and whether they were met. Also, they address the observation of caring behaviors and service learning activities. I am able to respond more effectively via email than in the hurried clinical setting during post conference.

Each student must self evaluate themselves at mid semester and end of semester. Faculty also evaluates and we sit down and compare evaluations and discuss progress or lack thereof.

I have instituted a means by which [students] peer evaluate things like head to toe assessments and give feedback rather than me grade or evaluate each one each week.

Faculty respondents clearly recognized the importance of providing meaningful feedback to students in order to optimize their clinical learning. Certainly, streamlining assignments and providing opportunities for students to develop their abilities to give and receive peer feedback are promising strategies to be further investigated. It is troubling, however, that many respondents recounted spending so little time providing feedback to students during a clinical day, and that on some clinical days students did not receive feedback directly from their instructor at all. The use of technology (e.g., email, online journals) may help faculty provide more feedback to students (Dugan, Wieland, & Hierholzer, 2008), but one wonders if this is an adequate substitute for feedback that occurs during clinical time and at the point of care (Clynes & Raftery, 2008). Moreover, the extent to which faculty can ensure that journaling captures clinically significant patient assessments, insights (or lack of insight) into a patient's concerns, and potential oversights (or errors or misunderstandings) — when it relies on what the student saw (not what was overlooked) and chooses to share — may limit the extent to which feedback on journal entries advances students' knowledge, skills, or attitudes. Research on the meaning and significance of various kinds and timing of feedback and its effect on students' clinical learning and performance is sorely needed.

Managing clinical teaching responsibilities with other expectations.

Nearly 25 percent of faculty respondents identified *managing clinical teaching responsibilities with other expectations of the faculty role* as one of the five most significant challenges, and 152 identified it as the most significant challenge they faced in their efforts to optimize students' clinical experiences. Fewer faculty shared the most important strategy they used to deal with this challenge than they did with the other four challenges in the top five. Of those who did address this challenge, most used the opportunity to explain the challenge more fully, frequently stating that they had not yet found a way to address it (e.g., "have not found a workable strategy yet"). Two participants even shared that addressing this challenge was "impossible." Sadly, many respondents were either in the process of leaving their position as a clinical teacher for "another job" or for "retirement" or were anticipating doing so, or referred to merely "surviving" or "persevering."

> Juggling all of the clinical and classroom teaching responsibilities along with committee participation, student advisory responsibilities, and professional/educational expectations have contributed to my "burnout" as a nursing faculty member. I am leaving nursing education at the end of the semester.

I haven't quite figured it out yet and I have resigned my full time faculty position to work in acute care...

I work longer hours and harder...to get everything done. As I get older, I think more about less clinical hours and possible retirement.

Managing clinical teaching responsibilities with other expectations of faculty role is my biggest challenge. I do not have a specific strategy other than just do it.

[*Managing clinical teaching responsibilities with other expectations is*] difficult... without feeling overwhelmed and fatigued. [I] work long hours preparing lecture material, both classroom and lab. [I'm] required to belong to several committees and also doing community work. [I] teach 18 contact hours. [I] haven't found a strategy that is effective as of yet. [I'm] looking for suggestions.

Unfortunately, I personally haven't figured out how to address [this challenge] effectively at this point in time. In particular — the demands of a tenure track faculty role alongside the demands of clinical teaching assignments with ever-increasing numbers of students is proving to be simply impossible.

Although some respondents indicated that they were "attempting to become more organized and use time better" as a way to address the challenge of managing multiple expectations, such statements were rare. The most common strategy reported for addressing this challenge was to "put in long hours over the 40 hour week" or to "simply... take work home."

I now simply expect to carry work home to complete on my leisure time on a regular basis, as there are not enough hours in a work day to meet all the faculty responsibilities. A clinical day involves about 9 straight hours, so all the clinical paperwork comes home with me to be reviewed/graded in the evening so that it can be returned to students the next day. Given students on multiple units, I spend time moving between the units, (time that used to be available to review their paperwork) but, given the numbers of students, I need to use multiple units. Since I may have 5 hours in the classroom on the days before and after clinicals, often after a clinical day, I need to return to the school anyway to get all the teaching materials together (like handouts, quizzes, etc.) ready for 0800 classes, extending that 9 hour day to a 10 or 11 hour day. Then there's all the committee work and meetings, the advisees to see, and countless other responsibilities involved in coordinating a course. Writing new lectures, researching evidence-based, best practices and continuously incorporating new information into lectures have become tasks that I perform when on vacation time as it's the only time left that's not already full of work- related items. The faculty role has become minimally a 60 hour a week endeavor. I'm not sure I can even call this a strategy, rather it's the only solution I can see.

I find that I use the evenings and weekends (that I am not teaching) to look after the other requirements of my position.

I don't get enough sleep — I work out of my house A LOT to get everything done.

In addition to the personal sacrifices, for some respondents the demands of clinical teaching resulted in sacrifices in their teaching, for example, "limiting the amount of time I spend on preparation for and evaluation of clinical work." Others shared how they "put less energy into clinical teaching," "read through students' paperwork at a much faster pace than I have done in the past," and had learned to "settle for 'good enough'" in their teaching.

For some, *managing clinical teaching responsibilities with other expectations* involved "learning to say no" or "refusing to take on more than a full load." For others, consulting with "more experienced faculty to get ideas about how to manage time in the clinical setting" or integrating their research and clinical teaching responsibilities was helpful.

Overall, the comments offered by respondents in relation to this challenge reflected an intensity not evidenced in responses to other challenges, even those marked by frustration as previously described. Indeed, the responses to this challenge suggested a "ripple effect" with ways in which other barriers and challenges were being addressed. For instance, *lack of quality clinical sites, size of clinical groups, and restrictions on the numbers of students or limitations to students' experiences imposed by clinical agencies* often resulted in faculty's being responsible for students on multiple units; this added to the workload of faculty as they "spen[t] time moving between units" — time that had been previously available to provide *appropriate guidance and supervision and meaningful feedback to students* and to cultivate relationships with staff nurses who are so critical to students' clinical learning. Similarly, because this time was not available for providing *appropriate guidance* and *meaningful feedback*, respondents' nonclinical time, together with evenings and weekends, became time to complete these responsibilities.

The lack of strategies offered by respondents, coupled with the number of respondents indicating that they were leaving clinical teaching or contemplating doing so as a result of the challenge of *managing clinical teaching responsibilities with other expectations of the faculty role*, suggests a dire need for the discipline to develop and test ways to effectively address this challenge. Investigating best practices of faculty preparation, development, and ongoing support would be valuable in this regard.

In addition, the effects of strategies devised to address other barriers and challenges must be evaluated for their effects not only on students' learning and readiness for practice, but also on faculty workload and satisfaction. Many of the strategies and issues that were shared require faculty to increase the hours they spend on completing what is needed for student learning, potentially putting them at even more risk for burnout. Given the persistent shortage of faculty nationally, we can ill afford to champion strategies that adversely affect clinical faculty's work life and abilities to teach and supervise students providing care. These concerns also apply to the staff nurses and preceptors involved in clinical education.

Supervising students' skill performance.

Nearly 25 percent of faculty respondents identified *supervising students' skill performance* as one of the five most significant challenges they faced, and 173 identified it as their most significant challenge in optimizing students' clinical learning. This finding was expected, given that more than 50 percent of respondents reported spending over 50 percent of their clinical time with students supervising skills. As with other challenges, some respondents described their efforts to manage the demands of skill supervision by better organizing their time, creating "checklists" or "clinical worksheets," being "better prepared for clinical," or using "better time management strategies."

By far the most common strategies respondents reported using to address this challenge were decreasing the number of skills or the number of students needing supervision during a clinical shift or having staff nurses, preceptors, assistants, or other students supervise skill performance.

Decreasing the number of skills or the number of students performing each skill.

Although many respondents spoke in general of decreasing the number of skills students were expected to perform, many focused specifically on medication administration. The difficulty in supervising this skill is exacerbated because of the sheer number of medications that each patient assigned to each student requires and the narrow window of time within which this skill must be accomplished. Many participants described using strategies directed specifically at decreasing the number of students expected to administer medications or perform other skills even though they recognized the limitations of this approach.

Supervising students' skill performance can take most of the day. I supervise half the group giving meds most of the morning and then have to give time to the other half of the group. [This is] no solution, just doing.

In my setting, I am the only one who can watch students pass meds. The students are so slow in this very first semester and we really need to be sure they are doing it correctly…So as a result I can only pass meds with 2-4 students a day. This means that students only get to pass meds twice in a semester. I guess it works out because it gives them a foundation and then in the next semester they can pass meds each week with the RN on the floor. The trouble is that I end up spending 2 out of [the] 5 hours we have in clinical passing meds and can't help with other things during that time.

Each clinical day, 2 students of 7 are chosen to administer medications. This is a Fundamentals class and the students are only on the floor for 5 hours. This strategy allows me to spend quality time with the 2 chosen students.

[I] pick 4 out of 8 students to perform medication administration each clinical [day] instead of trying to keep up with all 8 each day.

I have decided many days to provide only some skills for students [to] experience [and] then forfeit the others so they can be done by the nurse in a more timely manner.

I assign a day for maybe two students to be "active" and they give medications and do skills. Each student gets their days.

I have not figured out a way to make this smoother. It takes way too much time to try and have 8 students pass meds on 2 patients each.

Other respondents decreased the types of medications that students would be expected to administer, in addition to decreasing the number of students administering them.

While working on a surgical unit, my 8 students each have many IV medications. There is no way that I can be with 8 students and get all the IV meds hung at 09:00 and still do dressing changes and packing. Therefore, I only allow 5 students to give meds on any one clinical day. The other three will continue to do patient care and skills but not the time consuming IV push or piggyback meds.

One participant described alternating the students administering medications within a single clinical shift to allow more students to demonstrate this skill during each clinical experience while ensuring the timely administration of medication.

[I] buddy two students and alternate their med administration. [I] allow two students to give meds at each hour so more students can give them [each shift] without affecting the scheduled time for administration.

Another common way faculty addressed the challenge of *supervising students' skill performance* was to decrease the number of students needing supervision by providing alternative experiences for some students in the clinical group.

I have a rotation of two students going to the OR and two to three students shadowing a nurse on another unit, then I can focus more time on the other three to four students on supervising their assessment and physical examination skills with the patient.

I try very hard to prioritize the time and activities of the day, while providing each student with "some semblance" of an effective experience. More and more with the acuity increasing, and the students not being ready to meet the challenge, I end the day feeling harried and ineffectual. [I] am very concerned about safety! The tool I use most to address this [challenge] is sending some [students] off the unit to observe elsewhere for the day, hoping it does meet some of their educational needs.

Students complete an observation day during the rotation. They also have a day assigned to the trauma nurse who floats the hospital. I stagger these days so that the number of students on the unit [is] decreased. I supervise the remaining students on the unit.

I send two students for an observation on a related floor. Each student then presents to the rest of the group their experiences. This allows me to then concentrate my energies on the remaining 8.

Other participants reported decreasing the number of patients or the complexity of patients assigned to students in order to facilitate supervision.

[I] assign less complex clients so I am not overwhelmed with student-patient experience and can assist and teach. [I assign] multiple students per patient so we can work together and [I can] teach skills two at a time.

I used to be able to assign students 2-3 patients [each]. Now, due to acuity of patients, lack of preparation academically of students, staff and agency regulations as well as my own age, I can't do it and provide the supervision that these students now require. I have to divide up the multiple patient assignments so that I no longer have 14 patients but 10 at the most. This does not give the student many chances to have multiple patients and have opportunities to organize an assignment effectively.

Again, it is important to interpret these findings carefully, remembering that the only insight into the strategies described is the few lines that respondents offered in response to the survey question. Nonetheless, the sheer frequency with which respondents reported decreasing the number of students completing skills during a clinical experience raises important questions for further investigation. For instance, is skill performance in a clinical setting essential in order for new nurses to effectively enter practice? Which skills are critical? What/how much skill performance must occur in the clinical setting, and what/how much can just as effectively occur outside the clinical environment? How many times must a skill be demonstrated for faculty to be assured that the student can perform it competently when the situation demands? How long does such competency last? And what skill repertoire do health care institutions expect new graduate nurses to demonstrate? Answers to these questions may provide important evidence of the extent to which faculty should continue the use of strategies directed toward decreasing the skills covered in clinical or the number of students completing them.

Also noteworthy is the frequency with which students are given observation experiences in lieu of more traditional clinical experiences (providing patient care) so that faculty members have fewer students to supervise. Although this is clearly a common strategy, it is uncertain how such experiences contribute to students' learning. Research that demonstrates the pedagogical value of such experiences and the requisite timing, duration, and debriefing to achieve this learning through such experiences is imperative.

Having staff nurses or preceptors supervise students' skill performance.

Although rarely, participants mentioned hiring "part-time, contractual, and/or in-house staff for the hospitals we are affiliated with to have students… perform skills and [be] supervised carefully," decreasing the size of clinical groups (e.g., from 12 students to 8 students per instructor), or using student assistants (more experienced prelicensure students, student peers, or graduate students) to assist with skill supervision. Indeed, using teaching assistants was also identified as a strategy for addressing the barrier presented by the size of clinical group, although as previously noted this strategy was not among the top three. Nonetheless, this was the most effective strategy used by respondents to address the barrier of size of clinical group. In addition to the strategies of hiring staff or using teaching assistants and decreasing the size of clinical groups, participants recounted using existing faculty differently. For instance, one participant reported having the "skills [lab] instructor" come to the clinical unit to check students off on skills, presumably freeing up the clinical instructor for other teaching activities. By far most commonly, however, faculty respondents' efforts were to enlist the assistance of staff nurses and preceptors to supervise students' skill performance.

I have gotten assistance from the nurses to supervise students' skills when I am busy with another student. This has worked well. It is a challenge to meet both the students' and staff's needs.

We have to rely on preceptors and the agency staff a lot to monitor the students and provide the instructors with feedback.

I will either have the staff nurse supervise [the student's skill performance] if I am busy or lose the skill if they are not willing or able to [do this].

The student is paired with the staff nurse assigned to the patient. The staff nurse acts as a preceptor when I am busy with another student. In this way the student does not miss any learning opportunities.

As with the strategies that respondents described for addressing other challenges, reliance on staff nurses or preceptors to assist with clinical teaching was often mentioned. The literature reflects a persistent effort to investigate how preceptors can be recruited, prepared, and retained/rewarded (Brammer, 2006; Lillibridge, 2007; Tilley et al., 2007; Udlis, 2008). Faculty respondents were clear that the use of staff and/or preceptors was an important resource for student learning. As the nursing shortage continues, the number of students increases, and health care organizations face difficult economic times, the reliance on this resource may be precarious. Moreover, the relationships, which must be cultivated, negotiated, and nurtured between instructors and staff nurses, may be jeopardized as a result of faculty supervising students across numerous clinical units and not having the time required to establish or maintain these bonds. The development and testing of new clinical models that increase the supervision and feedback given to students and maximize students' learning from expert staff nurses — while decreasing the burden on faculty, staff, and preceptors — is certainly a priority for future research.

Despite the use of these strategies, faculty respondents commonly remarked about the difficulty that *supervising students' skill performance* presents.

This is a constant problem. I have increased my clinical hours without compensation to handle this problem.

[*Supervising students' skill performance*] is very hard. [I'm] still working on this. [I] run my legs off [and] try not to miss an opportunity, do some skills reviews prior to clinical.

The unpredictability of events on a hospital unit sometimes makes it difficult for me to supervise students as much as I would like.

When I started working here 11 years ago we did not have any preceptored clinicals. Now the entire second year (with the exception of the management clinical) is preceptored. We did not use any clinical simulations, but now we have simulations in both the lab and virtually. The clinical agencies did not have such strict limits on the number of students that we can take to a particular floor. All of our major or clinical courses were team taught with 2 or 3 faculty members working together. Now the majority of them are taught by 1 faculty. Eleven years ago we did not utilize any teaching assistants (ADN or BSN prepared RNs) or part time instructors. Now we average 5 teaching assistants and are employing 5 part time MSN prepared faculty. We have had two full time positions vacant since May of this year.

Respondents' references to decreasing the number of skills and the number of students performing them, as well as the use of staff nurses or preceptors to supervise students' skill performance, were both common and consistent. Noticeably absent was any description of the kinds of learning made possible by a decrease in the number of skills students perform, although alternatives are beginning to appear in the nursing literature. For instance, Lasater and Nielsen (2009) studied the effect of faculty's shifting attention from total patient care and the performance of the associated skills to concept-based clinical learning activities. Findings suggest that the use of concept-based learning activities deepens students' clinical thinking and abilities to make sound clinical judgments. Similar efforts were described by Giddens and colleagues (2008). Continued investigation into such emerging approaches to clinical education and their effects on student learning over time is critical to the widespread use of new clinical models. Also absent was any mention of how staff nurses and preceptors are prepared to be instructors and utilize principles of learning when working with students. As previously mentioned, being a good clinician does not necessarily equate to being a good educator (Brammer, 2006). Best practices for teaching and learning are needed in order to optimize student learning.

Overall, the strategies that respondents identified as the single most important strategy they used to address a particular challenge were rated as somewhat effective to effective. What remains unclear is how respondents conceptualized effectiveness. In other words, it seems probable that these strategies are effective at making the current model of clinical education more manageable (e.g., decreasing the number of students/skills that a single faculty member supervises), even if not optimal, but how effective are these strategies in promoting students' learning? How has the widespread use of these strategies influenced students' readiness for and transition into practice? How sustainable are these approaches? Clearly, issues around supervising students' skill performance remain priorities for research.

Discussion

The findings from this study highlight the barriers and challenges that faculty face when teaching in clinical settings in prelicensure RN programs.

Although respondents identified and described each barrier and challenge separately, it is noteworthy that most of these are closely connected. For example, the lack of quality clinical sites was identified by respondents as the most significant barrier they faced in their efforts to optimize students' learning in clinical settings. This finding is not surprising in light of the persistent demand for schools to admit, educate, and graduate more students, more quickly, to ease the shortage of nurses nationally. Although faculty reported employing a wide range of strategies to address this barrier, most of these strategies were perceived to be only minimally to somewhat effective. In addition, throughout the survey it became apparent that the strategies employed to address one barrier (e.g., the lack of quality clinical sites) frequently created and/ or exacerbated other problems that were equally difficult for faculty to address (e.g., providing appropriate guidance and supervision; providing meaningful feedback to students).

These findings support the contention that the traditional model of clinical education is no longer effective (Tanner, 2006a) but that it has not been altered substantially for decades (MacIntyre, Murray, Teel, & Karshmer, 2009). While the acuity of patients in the hospital and in nursing homes, clinics, private homes, and other health care settings has increased, our model of clinical education has not changed accordingly. Indeed, the majority of faculty responses to these common barriers and challenges demonstrate that substantial effort is being made by faculty to sustain a model of clinical education that may now be obsolete and ineffective at best, and counterproductive at worst, given the current context of health care. For example, the use of staff nurses and preceptors was a strategy that faculty frequently reported using to deal with a number of challenges. In some cases, staff nurses and preceptors were used by faculty as a stop-gap strategy to provide supervision when the faculty member was not immediately available because of the large number of students to be supervised or the dispersion of students across multiple units. In other cases, it was a longer-term strategy whereby "stronger students" worked with staff nurses or preceptors to allow the faculty member to provide more supervision and guidance to "weaker students."

The sheer frequency of the use of staff nurses and preceptors as noted by faculty respondents is troublesome in terms of how these clinicians were used, as well as in terms of the sustainability of this strategy for optimizing students' clinical learning. That is, references to the use of staff nurses and/or preceptors suggest that often, when the work of clinical teaching became overwhelming for faculty members, some of this work was shifted to these clinical experts. The literature shows that staff nurses' priority is patient care, not student learning, and they are already working faster and harder than employees in other industries (Lindberg, Nash, & Lindberg, 2008). Adding the responsibility of supervising students to this complex work is a risky strategy as a stop-gap measure, particularly during difficult economic times when some organizations are cutting back on staffing and other resources that previously supported the additional work of student supervision. This strategy is also problematic because, again, good clinicians are not necessarily good educators (Brammer, 2006) since they may be unfamiliar with the theoretical underpinnings of the curriculum and have difficulty bridging theory and practice. Clinicians often do not have qualifications beyond their initial general preparation (Altmann, 2006), and they may feel unprepared for (Jacobson & Grindel, 2006) and overwhelmed by the additional responsibilities of educating students.

Moreover, many respondents, despite having an average of more than 12 years of experience teaching in clinical settings, described how overwhelming it was to supervise students in complex clinical settings marked by high patient acuity and rapid turnover. Shifting the work of clinical teaching to staff nurses or preceptors — many of whom have little teaching experience and no background knowledge of the curriculum, each student's skill and experience level, or evidence-based pedagogies — may fail to optimize students' learning. This shifting creates haphazard learning environments for students and unpredictable environments for staff nurses (who can be called upon at any time to supervise a student they may or may not know), and it may well lead to incivility on the part of staff nurses and preceptors, to "burnout," and/or to inability or unwillingness to take on the additional work of student supervision.

It is time for widespread research and development of long-term, sustainable, effective models of clinical education — models that address the common barriers and challenges to optimizing clinical learning without further straining limited resources (faculty, clinical sites, and staff nurses and preceptors). This development will rely on the differentiation of critical clinical experiences, meaning those encounters with patients that are crucial in order for students to learn the practice of nursing, from the experiences that contribute to students' clinical practice but that can occur in a simulation lab, classroom, or other venue. Similarly, identifying what aspects of clinical learning are best taught, reinforced, and/or supervised by faculty members and what aspects are best handled by expert clinicians while care is being provided could guide the development of more effective and sustainable clinical education models (Connolly & Wilson, 2008; MacIntyre et al., 2009). Perhaps we are overusing limited clinical sites to provide experiences that could be more effectively offered in other ways and underusing the expertise of staff nurses when they are merely "filling in" for supervision that a faculty member is not able to provide.

In addition, attention to the role expectations for faculty and staff nurses is critical to the development of new clinical models. MacIntyre and colleagues (2009) suggest a reconceptualization of the roles of clinical faculty and staff nurses engaged in clinical teaching and of the relationships that students have with staff nurses. Such reconceptualization could foster students' abilities to build professional relationships with expert nurses over time because the student would have more ready access to the staff nurses' expertise without the faculty member's acting as intermediary. In addition, this role reconceptualization could foster staff nurses' abilities to get to know and connect with students to provide more individualized and situation-specific guidance. Dedicated education units (Moscato et al., 2007), in which students are assigned to a staff nurse rather than to a patient and staff nurses intentionally develop one-on-one relationships with students over the course of an entire term, or longer, is one promising model that merits further investigation.

Respondents' descriptions of the challenge of skill supervision and their attempts to address it suggest that this is another critical area for investigation. Faculty respondents identified the challenge of supervising students' skill performance as the most time-consuming aspect of teaching in clinical settings; and more than 50 percent of respondents who identified this as the most time-consuming aspect of their role reported that such supervision absorbed more than 50 percent of their time in clinical. In general, faculty respondents reported addressing this challenge by decreasing the number of skills students perform; using preceptors, staff nurses, graduate assistants, or other students to assist with skill supervision; and/or decreasing the size of the group of students to be supervised by creating alternative experiences for some students in the group (such as observation experiences). Determining critical learning encounters that promote students' learning in clinical settings, as well as identifying what is best learned in the clinical setting versus what can be learned in a simulation lab or other setting, is imperative if this challenge is to be successfully addressed.

For instance, many faculty respondents reported drastically decreasing the number of students performing particular skills (such as administering medications) during a clinical experience and/or pairing students to provide care to a single patient. It was interesting, in light of this challenge, that no respondents suggested reevaluating the skills students are required to perform, the number of required clinical hours necessary for learning or demonstrating their competency with these skills, or the way in which students spend time in clinical settings (and its effect on their learning). For example, it could be argued that our traditional approach to teaching medication administration is not effective, as medication errors continue to occur, and at alarming rates, in contemporary health care settings (Institute of Medicine, 2007). In addition, the safety literature clearly demonstrates that improvements in patient safety require the recognition of systems issues that influence the risk of error rather than an isolated focus on errors committed by individual clinicians. Thus, the overwhelming focus on medication administration not only absorbs an inordinate amount of clinical time but may not, in fact, improve patient safety at all and may inadvertently contribute to the problem as new nurses are erroneously socialized to equate the repetition of this skill with continuing competency in practice (Ironside, 2008). In addition, even though many faculty described how supervising students' skill performance (particularly medication administration) overtook their available clinical time and noted how frequently their interaction with students was severely limited (even, at times, absent), the model being used was not questioned. In all but a few cases, decreasing the number of skills or the number of students performing them was cited as a way to address the problems of supervision while retaining the same model of clinical education that created the problems in the first place. Rarely did respondents characterize using these strategies (decreasing the number of skills to be supervised or the numbers of students performing them) as an opportunity to engage students in the higher-level thinking that occurs in clinical settings, such as making qualitative distinctions among patients with similar conditions, experiences, or symptom presentation or picking up on nuanced changes in patient states.

Perhaps nowhere are the problems with the predominant model of clinical education more apparent than with skill supervision. This model perpetuates a technical conceptualization of students' clinical experience, which is apparent in the organization of clinical experiences in terms of required hours, checklists of the skills that must be learned and demonstrated, and the ubiquitous focus on total patient care during every clinical experience. It is noteworthy that when deficits are identified in students' readiness for practice, both faculty and students frequently express the desire for more clinical experience (Dahlberg, Ekebergh, & Ironside, 2003). In most cases, the desire for more assumes more of the same — more hours, more skills, and more experience providing total patient care. Indeed, many programs are encouraging students to complete summer internships or residencies. Although these programs may well be important to students as they transition into patient care, how can the "lessons learned" from these programs be leveraged to reshape basic nursing education? Could clinical models be developed that integrate the best practices of internship or residency models throughout nursing education?

Research investigating the kinds of experiences students have in clinical settings and the ways in which these experiences influence their readiness for practice is also imperative. It is time to rigorously investigate the relationship between skill performance and students' readiness for and integration into professional practice. Given the current context of care, what skills are required for generalist practice and what skills are no longer relevant? Are there skills that we should *no longer teach* as part of prelicensure education? Could limiting the focus on traditional skill performance (associated with total patient care) create other opportunities for faculty and/or staff nurses to work with students to develop their situated thinking and reasoning skills, their ability to make sound clinical judgments, and their ability to work collaboratively with an interdisciplinary team?

The widespread use of observation experiences raises similar questions. Faculty respondents frequently identified sending students to observe the nursing care being provided in another area, or a nurse functioning in another role, as a mechanism for making the current model of clinical education manageable. Such strategies are typically justified as assisting students to appreciate the different contexts in which nurses work or to explore the possibilities for their future employment. Certainly decreasing the number of students in a clinical group (using the traditional model) helps the faculty member attend to the learning of the remaining, smaller group of students. What is the cost to the students sent on observational experiences? This is not to suggest that all observational experiences are ineffective or that no learning can occur during these experiences, but it is concerning that so little evidence exists to support this common practice. It is time to question the utility of such experiences and to investigate the ways in which they contribute to or perhaps interrupt students' opportunities to establish sustained relationships with staff nurses on particular clinical units, to take on multiple patient assignments or assignments involving more complex patients, to investigate the influence of the systems in which care is provided, and so on. Again, documenting the learning that these experiences foster, the timing of this learning, and the impact of this learning on readiness for practice is an important area for future inquiry.

The need for new pedagogies and models of clinical education has perhaps never been greater. Although important work is occurring in this area, it is largely underfunded, underdisseminated, and underutilized. Even many of the most common strategies described in this survey (such as providing observation experiences) remain undertheorized and untested. The respondents' descriptions of the barriers and challenges they face and the strategies they use to address them suggest that faculty are expending tremendous efforts to sustain a failing model of clinical education, at great expense to themselves (and over the long term to the discipline as clinical faculty leave teaching to assume other positions) and to student learning. Further development and rigorous testing of nursing pedagogies and clinical models are crucial to the identification of best practices in teaching and learning in clinical settings.

Progress in the development and testing of new models for clinical education is hampered by (a) the lack of faculty, staff nurses, and preceptors prepared for the faculty role; (b) the low levels of pedagogical literacy among faculty; (c) the lack of faculty prepared to conduct large-scale multisite, methodologically sophisticated studies of nursing education; and (d) the lack of substantive funding to support this work.

The Need for Faculty Preparation

The findings of this study suggest that preparation for teaching in clinical settings must be widely available to faculty, staff nurses and preceptors, and teaching assistants. The complexity of current health care environments requires those who teach in clinical settings to be adept at using evidence-based pedagogies to create learning encounters that develop students' clinical discernment, reasoning, and judgment in an intentional way. Knowledge of the practice of nursing is insufficient, as is knowledge of teaching principles or learning theories alone. Teaching in clinical settings will require an exquisite integration of both, and faculty preparation programs must provide this integration. Practicum experiences wherein new faculty, staff nurses and preceptors, and teaching assistants hone their skills at using these pedagogies to optimize student learning may well accelerate the development, use, and testing of new clinical models.

Low Levels of Pedagogical Literacy

Throughout the survey, respondents described strategies they used to address the most significant barriers and challenges that they faced. In all but a few cases, these strategies reflected the perpetuation of the current model of clinical education, and they were most commonly described by faculty as only minimally to somewhat effective. The current context of health care, the shortage of faculty, and the persistent problems with the traditional model of clinical education (one faculty member supervising a group of up to 10 students who each provide total patient care to one or two patients) require that new, research-based pedagogies be developed and enacted — pedagogies that are responsive to the context in which teaching and learning occur and the unique opportunities for and challenges to learning that arise in clinical settings. New pedagogies will assist faculty to overcome the conventional emphasis on cognitive gain and skill acquisition and the assumption of the direct and corresponding relationship between classroom and clinical learning to embrace more porous boundaries between the kinds of learning that occur across settings. For instance, new pedagogies can provide the opportunities for students to investigate nursing phenomena during clinical experiences, as well as to explore their assumptions and the patient experiences that accompany particular conditions or situations. Such discussions can further shape those occurring in classrooms, experiences in simulation labs, and so forth. Faculty development programs, as well as teacher preparation programs, must assist faculty to investigate, develop, use, and evaluate diverse pedagogies to optimize student learning.

Lack of Faculty Prepared to Conduct Research in Nursing Education

With the advent of national-level funding for nursing research in clinical practice, the preparation of nurses to conduct research in nursing education became largely underfunded and undervalued. Most schools of nursing did not allow doctoral students to conduct studies of nursing education, and many new faculty members were encouraged to pursue clinical lines of inquiry, rather than inquiry into teaching and learning, in order to achieve tenure and promotion in rank. The outcome of these efforts is that research in many clinical areas has flourished and the science of nursing has become well articulated, while the science of nursing education has failed to keep pace with developments in the field. Though many doctoral programs are now supporting the preparation of researchers in nursing education, the pool of senior faculty with expertise in developing and sustaining a program of research in nursing education is exceedingly small. As a result, the evidence base for how students can best be prepared for practice, particularly in clinical settings, is narrowly conceptualized and extremely limited in depth, breadth, and methodological sophistication. This contributes to the perpetuation of traditional educational practices (despite the documented problems) and the lack of established best practices for clinical education. It is time for the discipline to create a strong network of support to advance the science of nursing education through the provision of funded training programs that connect senior researchers to those seeking preparation in the conduct of such research (Broome, 2009). Furthermore, how students are prepared for and integrated into practice has such serious ramifications that it is, perhaps, timely for *all* doctoral students to take required coursework in nursing pedagogies and to conduct studies to evaluate their use in a variety of settings as part of their research training.

Lack of Funding for Research in Nursing Education

Advancing the science of nursing education related to students' learning in clinical settings is imperative to ensure that future pedagogical decisions are evidence based and that our educational practices keep pace with the rapidly changing field in which students learn. Substantive, methodologically sophisticated, longitudinal research is desperately needed. In order for this to happen, the national-level funding agencies and foundations must target money for the development and testing of pedagogically sophisticated models of clinical education and the evaluation of such preparation on students' readiness for and integration into practice, as well as on the quality of care provided by graduates. It is shortsighted to assume that evidence from the best, most rigorous clinical nursing studies can influence patient care without a nurse (and other well-trained health care professionals) at the bedside who has been well prepared to utilize that science and evaluate its effect on particular patient encounters. Funding demonstration projects of pedagogical reform would further provide for the rigorous testing and comparison of diverse pedagogical models to show how these influence students' readiness for and integration into practice, as well as how this preparation affects the quality of patient care.

Limitations

One limitation of the present study is that it used a convenience sample. Survey respondents self-selected, and the extent to which this sample represents the population of clinical faculty is unknown. A further limitation is the use of open-ended items, with respondents asked to enter the top five challenges from the list provided and to describe a single strategy they used to address one of these challenges. Many of the responses were very brief, yielding little insight into the strategy, how it was used, or in what ways it was or was not effective. Also, some respondents entered challenges that were not on the list provided, and others failed to describe a strategy at all and instead offered further description of the challenge. As previously discussed, at times the relationship between the strategy described and the challenge it was purported to address was unclear. These factors limit the analysis of data and increase the risk that the investigators misunderstood the intent of a respondent's comment. Lastly, this study was limited in the investigators' ability to correlate the challenges and barriers faced, as well as the strategies used to address them, with specific program variables. Clearly there are many site-specific factors that influence the identification of barriers and challenges, the strategies that are available or possible for use in addressing them, and the perceptions or measures of effectiveness. Thus, the findings of this study should be interpreted with caution.

Recommendations

Congruent with the Blue Ribbon Panel's major areas of focus for future research in nursing education, this study further emphasizes the following needs:

- New clinical models must be developed and tested across sites, locations, types of programs, and levels of students. The influence of these models on students' learning and readiness for and integration into practice must be examined using multi-site, methodologically sophisticated studies. These models must foster partnerships among faculty, students, schools, clinical agencies, staff nurses and preceptors that align clinical learning with contemporary practice and health care needs.

- The pedagogical practices enacted by clinical teachers must be evidence-based, and the learning outcomes evaluated must be well defined, robust, and relevant to contemporary practice settings. In other words, we can no longer rely on NCLEX° pass rates, skill demonstrations, and the completion of required clinical hours and rotations as proxies for pedagogical effectiveness. Assessment of the effects of our pedagogical practices must also include investigation into the "dosage" of particular experiences, timing of these experiences, the duration of the desired effects, and so forth. The meaning and significance of these pedagogical practices to faculty, students, and staff nurses/preceptors must also be evaluated.

- Research is needed to differentiate the critical aspects of learning the practice of nursing that must occur in clinical settings from those that can be learned in classrooms, laboratories, simulation centers, or other venues. Such research must include evidence of the transferability of knowledge, skills, and attitudes from different nonclinical learning experiences (such as simulation experiences) to students' clinical practice, as well as the effect on the quality of care provided by students.

Teaching in clinical settings is demanding work, and participant responses to this survey attest to the valiant efforts of many clinical faculty members to optimize students' clinical learning despite significant obstacles. It seems clear that doing nothing — striving to find ways to save the traditional model of education — is not an option. We are reminded of the warning that Porter-O'Grady issued nine years ago for its continuing relevance to this discussion.

Holding on to old notions and practices that no longer characterize the demands of the time will do nothing but exacerbate the conditions which facilitate the demise of nurses and nursing work. (2001, p. 183)

The time to act has come. It is time to move beyond tradition, develop and use new pedagogies for clinical education, and support rigorous inquiry into the effects of this work on student preparation and on safe, quality patient care. Those for whom the students of today will care in the future deserve nothing less.

References

Altmann, T. K. (2006). Preceptor selection, orientation, and evaluation in baccalaureate nursing education. *International Journal of Nursing Education Scholarship, 3*(1), Article 1, 1-16.

American Organization of Nurse Executives (AONE). (2004). Position statement on pre-licensure supervised clinical instruction. Retrieved October 4, 2009, from http://www.aone.org/aone/advocacy/PositionStatementPre-licensureclinicalexperien ceformatted.pdf

Ard, N., Rogers, K., & Vinten, S. (2008). Summary of the survey on clinical education in nursing [Headlines from the NLN]. *Nursing Education Perspectives, 29*, 238-245.

Aston, L., & Molassiotis, A. (2003). Supervising and supporting student nurses in clinical placements: The peer support initiative. *Nurse Education Today, 23*, 202-210.

Benner, P., Sutphen, M., Leonard, V., & Day, L. (2009). *Educating nurses: A call for radical transformation.* San Francisco: Jossey-Bass.

Brammer, J. D. (2006). RN as gatekeeper: Student understanding of the RN buddy role in clinical practice experience. *Nurse Education Today, 26*, 697-704.

Broome, M. E. (2009). Building the science for nursing education: Vision or improbable dream [Editorial]. *Nursing Outlook, 57*, 177-179.

Clynes, M. P., & Raftery, S. E. C. (2008). Feedback: An essential element of student learning in clinical practice. *Nurse Education in Practice, 8*, 405-411.

Connolly, M. A., & Wilson, C. J. (2008). Revitalizing academic-service partnerships to resolve nursing faculty shortages. AACN *Advanced Critical Care, 19*(1), 85-97.

Cronenwett, L., Sherwood, G., Barnsteiner, J., Disch, J., Johnson, J., Mitchell, P., et al. (2007). Quality and safety education for nurses. *Nursing Outlook, 55*, 122-131.

Dahlberg, K., Ekebergh, M., & Ironside, P. M. (2003). Converging conversations from phenomenological pedagogies: Toward a science of health professions education. In N. Diekelmann & P. Ironside (Eds.), *Teaching practitioners of care: New pedagogies for the health professions* (Vol. 2, pp. 22-58). Madison, WI: University of Wisconsin Press.

Daley, L. K., Menke, E., Kirkpatrick, B., & Sheets, D. (2008). Partners in practice: A win-win model for clinical education. *Journal of Nursing Education, 47*, 30-32.

Diekelmann, N., & Diekelmann, J. (2009). *Schooling learning teaching: Toward narrative pedagogy*. New York: iUniverse.

Dugan, M. A., Wieland, D., & Hierholzer, R. (2008). Communicating clinical agency orientation materials via the university portal. *Nurse Educator, 33*, 241-243.

Giddens, J., Brady, D., Brown, P., Wright, M., Smith, D., & Harris, J. (2008). A new curriculum for a new era of nursing education. *Nursing Education Perspectives, 29*, 200-205.

Gubrud-Howe, P., Shaver, K. S., Tanner, C. A., Bennett-Stillmaker, J., Daidson, S. B., Flaherty-Robb, M., et al. (2003). A challenge to meet the future: Nursing education in Oregon, 2010. *Journal of Nursing Education, 42*, 163-167.

Gubrud, P., & Schoessler, M. (2009). OCNE clinical education model. In N. Ard & T. M. Valiga (Eds.). *Clinical nursing education: Current reflections* (pp. 39-58). New York: National League for Nursing.

Institute of Medicine. (2007). *Preventing medication errors*. Washington, DC: National Academies Press.

Ironside, P. M. (2001). Creating a research base for nursing education: An interpretive review of conventional, critical, feminist, postmodern, and phenomenologic pedagogies. *Advances in Nursing Science, 23*(3), 72-87.

Ironside, P. M. (2005). Teaching thinking and reaching the limits of memorization: Enacting new pedagogies. *Journal of Nursing Education, 44*, 441-449.

Ironside, P. M. (2006). Using narrative pedagogy: Learning and practicing interpretive thinking. *Journal of Advanced Nursing, 55*, 478-486.

Ironside, P. M. (2008). Safeguarding patients through continuing competency. *Journal of Continuing Education in Nursing, 390*, 92-94.

Jacobson, L., & Grindel, C. (2006). [Headlines from NLN.] What is happening in pre-licensure RN clinical nursing education? Findings from the Faculty and Administrator Survey on Clinical Nursing Education. *Nursing Education Perspectives, 27*(2), 108-109.

Lasater, K., & Nielsen, A. (2009). The influence of concept-based learning activities on students' clinical judgment development. *Journal of Nursing Education, 48*, 441-446.

Lillibridge, J. (2007). Using clinical nurses as preceptors to teach leadership and management to senior nursing students: A qualitative descriptive study. *Nurse Education in Practice, 7*, 44-52.

Lindberg, C., Nash, S., & Lindberg, C. (2008). *On the edge: Nursing in the age of complexity*. Bordentown, NJ: Plexus.

Luhanga, F., Yonge, O., & Myrick, F. (2008). Hallmarks of unsafe practice: What preceptors know. *Journal for Nurses in Staff Development, 24*, 257-264.

MacIntyre, R. C., Murray, T. A., Teel, C. S., & Karshmer, J. F. (2009). Five recommendations for prelicensure clinical nursing education. *Journal of Nursing Education, 48*, 447-453.

McNelis, A. M., & Ironside, P. M. (2009). National Survey on Clinical Education in Prelicensure Nursing Education Programs. In N. Ard & T. M. Valiga (Eds.), *Clinical nursing education: Current reflections* (pp. 25-38). New York: National League for Nursing.

Moscato, S. R., Miller, J., Logsdon, K., Weinberg, S., & Chorpenning, L. (2007). Dedicated education unit: An innovative clinical partner education model. *Nursing Outlook, 55*, 31-37.

National Council of State Boards of Nursing (NCSBN). (2005). Clinical instruction in prelicensure nursing programs [Position paper]. Retrieved from http://www.ncsbn.org/Final_Clinical_Instr_Pre_Nsg_program.pdf

Porter-O'Grady, T. (2001). Profound change: 21st century nursing. *Nursing Outlook, 49*(4), 182-186.

Scheckel, M. M., & Ironside, P. M. (2006). Enacting narrative pedagogy: Cultivating interpretive thinking. *Nursing Outlook, 54*, 159-165.

Secomb, J. (2007). A systematic review of peer teaching and learning in clinical education. *Journal of Clinical Nursing, 17*, 703-716.

Tanner, C. A. (2006a). The next transformation: Clinical education [Editorial]. *Journal of Nursing Education, 45*, 99-100.

Tanner, C. A. (2006b). Thinking like a nurse: A research-based model of clinical judgment in nursing. *Journal of Nursing Education, 45*, 204-211.

Tilley, D. S., Allen, P., Collins, C., Bridges, R. A., Francis, P., & Green, A. (2007). Promoting clinical competence: Using scaffolded instruction for practice-based learning. *Journal of Professional Nursing, 23*, 285-289.

Tobar, K., Wall, D., Parsh, B., & Sampson, J. (2007). Use of 12-hour clinical shifts in nursing education: Faculty, staff, and student response. *Nurse Educator 32*(5), 190-191.

Udlis, K. A. (2008). Preceptorship in undergraduate nursing education: An integrative review. *Journal of Nursing Education, 47*, 20-29.

Warner, J. R., & Moscato, S. R. (2009). Innovative approach to clinical education: Dedicated education units. In N. Ard & T. M. Valiga (Eds.). *Clinical nursing education: Current reflections* (pp. 59-70). New York: National League for Nursing.

Yonge, O. J., Anderson, M., Profetto-McGrath, J., Olson, J. K., Skillen, D. L., Boman, J., et al. (2005). An inventory of nursing education research. *International Journal of Nursing Education Scholarship, 2*(1), Article 11.